Horsewhip THE DOCTOR

Horsewhip THE DOCTOR

Tales from Our Medical Past

Ross Patrick

University of Queensland Press

ST LUCIA • LONDON • NEW YORK

First published 1985 by University of Queensland Press
Box 42, St Lucia, Queensland, Australia

Typeset by University of Queensland Press
Printed in Australia by Dominion Press — Hedges & Bell

Distributed in the UK and Europe by University of Queensland Press
Dunhams Lane, Letchworth, Herts. SG6 1LF England

Distributed in the USA and Canada by University of Queensland Press
5 South Union Street, Lawrence, Mass. 01843 USA

Cataloguing in Publication Data

National Library of Australia

Patrick, Ross, 1914-
Horsewhip the doctor.

1. Physicians - Queensland - Anecdotes, facetial, satire, etc. I. Title.

610.69'52'09943

Library of Congress

Patrick, Ross, 1914-

Horsewhip the doctor.

1. Physicians — Australia — History. 2. Medicine— Australia — History. I. Title.
R671.P38 1985 610'.92'4[B] 85-1015

ISBN 0 7022 1867 7

Contents

Illustrations

Acknowledgments

My wife Heather suggested that I write this book. Douglas Gordon, Emeritus Professor of Social and Preventive Medicine, Colin Sheehan, Oxley Librarian, and Paul Wilson, Queensland State Archivist, encouraged the project and suggested sources for material.

Help with individual narratives was given by Mary McCracken (nee Stewart-Kenny), Sir Abraham Fryberg, Dr Konrad Hirschfeld, Colleen Mellish, Caroline Nesbitt and Dr Aubrey Pye. Jack Dale assisted with the photography and Tim Moroney drew my attention to the cartoon on leprosy.

Courteous help was given by the staff of the following archives and libraries : The National Library of Ireland; Tasmanian Archives, Hobart; Latrobe Library, Melbourne; Mitchell Library and the Archives Office of New South Wales, Sydney; and the Queensland State Archives, Oxley Library and the Queensland Parliamentary Library, Brisbane.

Surgeon Sacked in Sex Scandal

> All the officers here are desperate grog-drinkers and cigar smokers except one other and myself. I have just now returned from a dinner party which Lieutenant Edwards gave in compliment to me, and at which all the officers were present except Mr Cowper, who, it seems, is greatly disliked. He is a most uncouth original, an excessive grog-drinker and smoker, and the most ill-tempered and quarrelsome man I ever saw, of which I witnessed repeated proofs already, though I am not yet a week at the settlement. However, I hope and confidently expect to act with such prudence in my intercourse with him as will prevent the possibility of any fracas between us. I really think he is half insane. However, he is aware of his dreadful temper, for he speaks about it and says he is quite sure he will yet be confined in a madhouse. He has some good points notwithstanding. I shall make you laugh by telling some anecdotes about him, please God.

These words formed part of a letter written by Assistant Surgeon J.F. Murray to his sister on 10 May 1830, a few days after he arrived at the Moreton Bay penal settlement. The man he was describing was Dr Henry Cowper, who had been sent as the first doctor to Moreton Bay in 1825. Henry Cowper was the son of Rev. William Cowper, who came to the colony of New South Wales in 1809, after being recruited as assistant chaplain by Rev. Samuel Marsden. Rev. Cowper later became Archdeacon of Cumberland. Henry Cowper was apprenticed to Dr William Redfern and helped his master in his practice and at the new Sydney Hospital in Macquarie Street. After three years' training with Redfern, the young Cowper was appointed assistant at the hospital. When he had completed two years' service in this position, he was regarded by Redfern as well-trained. A specially convened board of examiners accredited Cowper as Australia's first qualified practitioner to have received all his training in the colony. To this qualification, Cowper later added membership of the College of Surgeons when he went to London.

Although well-trained, Cowper was not an ideal employee whilst at Sydney Hospital. Evidence of misdemeanours committed by the young surgeon appear in the Report into the Colony of New South Wales written by J.T. Bigge, who was commissioned in 1819 by the British government to enquire into almost everything that went on in the colony. Unfavourable comments contained in Bigge's report (and found also in the Wentworth papers in the Mitchell Library, Sydney), include a complaint from Redfern that Cowper was ungrateful and of bad behaviour. It was alleged the young doctor was careless in keeping hospital records and neglected his duty by failing to supply medicine to Newcastle Hospital. At one stage, he was considered untrustworthy and he was kept on only out of respect for his father. He was further accused of supplying his friends with medicines, stockings, and other items from the hospital store. However, not all the reports were unfavourable. Bowman, the principal colonial surgeon, was quoted as saying in 1819 that "he has perfect knowledge of the hospital. If called to assist the clerk, his ingenuity would shine with true brightness".

Before Cowper arrived at Moreton Bay, the commissariat storeman acted as surgeon for the convicts and their keepers. When the doctor first came to the settlement there was no hospital. Through the efforts of Captain Logan, the best-known of the commandants at the penal settlement, a brick hospital was built in 1827 on the site now occupied by the Supreme Court, between what is now George Street and North Quay. Here, with the help of an untrained staff, some of whom were convicts, Cowper nursed the convict sick and an occasional ailing soldier. The diseases responsible for most of the admissions were eye disease, fever (probably malaria) and dysentery. The last condition had a high mortality due to the poor physical condition of the convicts, brought on by overcrowding, malnutrition and a low standard of hygiene. The only water supply was collected in ponds in wet weather and in the dry season the water became stagnant and unfit for use. Cowper's meticulously kept hospital records (still available in the Queensland State Archives) show that sickness and suffering reached a crescendo in the summer of 1828–29. During this period, there were over 100 patients in the small hospital every day. The maximum recorded was 181 patients, and the doctor was responsible for a number of outpatients as well. These came from a convict population of less than 1000. In 1829, 73 died in the hospital, mainly from dysentery and related diseases. Dr Cowper battled this epidemic with the drugs available in those days, few of them very effective. There were no sulpha drugs and no antibiotics. From available records it is clear that the medical care given by Cowper, with the facilities he had, was of a high standard. Evidence that he was more than a good clinical practitioner is seen in his report of an epidemiological survey he carried out, comparing the incidence of disease in the main settlement and in the outstation at Eagle Farm. None of the commandants under whom he served passed any adverse comment on his medical ability.

Cowper had other than purely medical duties. In a diary kept by Peter Spicer, the superintendent of convicts, a frequent entry was: "Yesterday, Sunday, the prisoners were mustered and inspected by the Superintendent and Divine Service was read to them by Dr Cowper". In February 1827, Logan told the colonial secretary in Sydney that "Mr Cowper has invariably read the funeral services at the interments which have taken place since my arrival at the settlement". There were not many deaths at that time, but, if this was still one of the doctor's duties during the dysentery epidemic of 1828–29, he must have been a busy man.

Towards the end of 1830, Logan went out on one of his numerous exploring trips, but failed to return to the main party. Several groups searched for him, but it was the party led by Dr Cowper which actually found Logan's body after he had been killed by the Aborigines. Captain Clunie, who had already arrived in Moreton Bay to relieve Logan, reported the incident and praised Cowper's efforts: "Hopes were still entertained of his [Logan's] being alive till the 28th ultimo, when Dr Cowper whose exertions on this occasion were very great and for which I felt indebted, discovered the dead horse stinking in a creek, and not far from it, at the top of the bank, the body of Captain Logan, buried about a foot underground".

During his time at Moreton Bay, Cowper made several trips to Sydney. He gave evidence in a murder trial and also appeared before an enquiry when Logan was accused of murder by the editor of the *Monitor*, E.S. Hall. Cowper told the enquiry that he attended punishments when more than fifty lashes were inflicted and that he inspected the backs of prisoners before and after flogging. Cowper's affidavit and evidence helped the enquiry conclude that the charges against Logan were unfounded. It was after his return from one of these trips that a scandal occurred which abruptly ended Cowper's career at Moreton Bay: an incident described by one author as an indiscretion and by another as a prank that went too far.

On this occasion, Dr Cowper had returned on the brig *Governor Phillip*. In the evening, he invited the vessel's master, Captain John Richards, to his residence next to the hospital. The doctor believed that, as there was another medical officer on the settle-

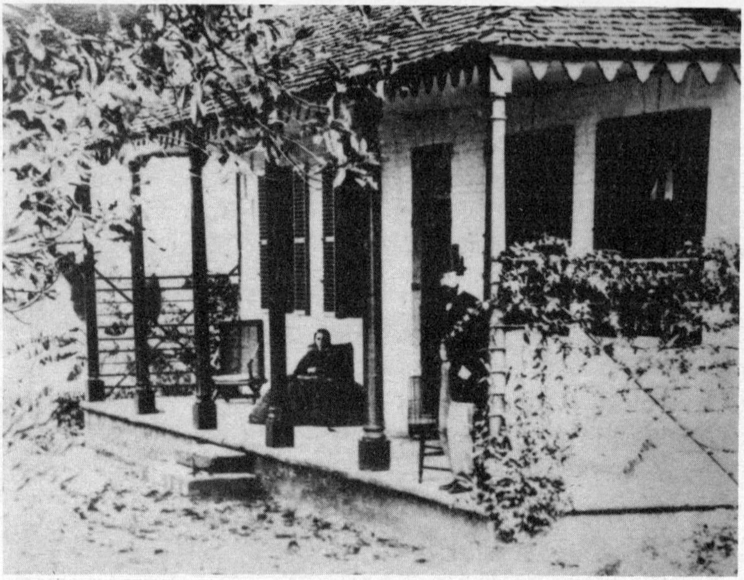

The surgeon's cottage, George Street — where the Supreme Court now stands — in 1862. (Courtesy AMA Queensland branch)

ment, he was entitled to indulge himself and his guest. So the two drank generously from the doctor's rum supply. Towards one o'clock in the morning, the two revellers decided to visit the inmates of the female factory. They took the hospital clerk, Halden, with them to carry a bottle of rum and four figs of tobacco. They climbed the high wall surrounding the factory and Richards spoke to the women in one of the rooms. They told him where a key to their room was secreted in the grounds and with this he opened the door. Richards shared the rum and their company until daylight. Meanwhile, Cowper — according to the subsequent enquiry — spoke through the window to women in another room but did not enter. It is believed that Constable Creedon, on duty at the factory, assisted in these activities. Towards dawn, Cowper persuaded Richards it was time to return to his residence. Had this been the end of the incident there would probably have been no sequence, for when Matron Blunt inspected the factory in the morning everything appeared in order. But two of the women, wishing the party to continue, pretended to be sick and were taken to the hospital. Cowper gave them more rum and one of them tried unsuccessfully to involve Richards in more frivolities. As they were being taken back to the factory one of them broke away from the escort and ran into the married soldiers' quarters. A corporal working in the garden was attracted to the scene and made a report to Captain Clunie, the commandant. Cowper gave contradictory statements to the commandant, partly to shield Richards and partly in his own defence. He also tried to persuade Private Blunt, the matron's husband, to give incorrect evidence, but the private was found drunk in Cowper's quarters and he, too, was in trouble.

Clunie set up a court of enquiry, consisting of Lieutenant Nagel as president, and Lieutenant Graham and Assistant Surgeon Murray as members. No doubt, in view of Murray's dislike of Cowper, it gave him some pleasure to sit in judgment of him. Clunie forwarded the report from the board of enquiry to the colonial secretary, Alexander McLeay, in Sydney. McLeay minuted the report and, submitting it to Governor Bourke, suggested the governor should take a lenient view of the incident:

> Mr Henry Cowper is the eldest son of the Revd. Wm. Cowper, Senior assistant chaplain, and has served in his present position 8 years without blame. Some allowance may perhaps be made for the circumstances of seclusion and privation in which officers are placed at Penal Settlements, rendering them both more liable to be unduly affected by convivial indulgence and more ready to avail themselves of it when opportunity offers. Whatever may be the degree of severity with which His Excellency might feel himself to visit the transaction viewed by itself, I do not think that the Service would suffer or any person either now or hereafter feel aggrieved if that severity were remitted on the express and avowed grounds of consideration for the long and faithful services of Mr Cowper's father.

Governor Bourke was not impressed by McLeay's minute and made his decision:

> After having given this case 24 hours consideration I can come to no other decision than that the principal delinquents, Cowper, Richards, Creedon and Halden be dismissed from their employment under the Colonial Government, and that Private Blunt of the 17th. Reg. be ordered back to his regimental duty and sent to Sydney by the first opportunity. It will be for Captain Clunie to consider whether after having removed her husband he can retain Mrs Blunt as Matron of the Factory. Nothing has appeared in the course of the investigation to incriminate her. Colonial Secretary will please to carry the foregoing instructions without delay.

When Principal Colonial Surgeon Bowman received a copy of this decision, he immediately wrote to the colonial secretary:

I have the honour to acknowledge the receipt of your letter of the 13th instant communicating that Mr Cowper, Assistant Surgeon at Moreton Bay shall be dismissed from his employment under the Colonial Government.

I regret exceedingly to learn that Mr Cowper should have conducted himself so indiscreetly after having served so many years at that settlement.

I beg leave to state for His Excellency's information that Mr Cowper is the son of one of the Senior Chaplains of the Colony and that he first commenced to study the Medical Profession at the General Hospital, Sydney some time previous to my being appointed to this department. Soon after my arrival here, he proceeded to England to complete his studies and having returned to the Colony received an appointment from Sir. Thos. Brisbane to the settlement at Moreton Bay, where he has continued to serve to the present time.

In the early period of that settlement Mr Cowper was subjected to many privations and had a very arduous duty to perform, in doing which he acquitted himself in such a manner as to deserve the approbation of his superiors and I believe this is the first complaint against him.

Under these circumstances I feel it my duty respectfully to request His Excellency to suspend his decision for the present and as Mr Cowper has conducted himself well eight years at that settlement, I may venture to hope his future conduct will merit the lenity His Excellency may now be pleased to extend to him.

Should His Excellency accede to my solicitation in favour of Mr Cowper, I would beg leave further to suggest that he be permitted to exchange duties with Mr Gamach at Norfolk Island, and by this arrangement he will be removed from his present connexions and be placed out of the way of temptation.

Governor Bourke was unmoved by this further pleading and Cowper left Moreton Bay settlement in disgrace. He returned south and entered private practice.

Death's Emigrant

In a quiet corner of the Dunwich cemetery on Stradbroke Island a modest headstone bears the inscription:

AROUND THIS STONE
ARE INTERRED
THE MORTAL REMAINS
OF
TWENTY-SIX EMIGRANTS
WHO
SEEKING IN THIS LAND
AN EARTHLY HOME
HAVE FOUND ELSEWHERE
WE TRUST
A BETTER COUNTRY

Simple metal markers indicate the individual graves. Nearby are the more substantial tombstones in memory of doctors David Ballow and George Mitchell. The memorials are grim reminders of a tragedy that occurred in 1850 when Ballow, Mitchell and the emigrants met their deaths.

David Keith Ballow was born at Montrose, County Angus on the east coast of Scotland on 27 October 1804. Graduating in medicine at Edinburgh University, he migrated to Sydney at the age of thirty. The gallant and jovial Scot married Margaret, youngest daughter of Captain Peter McArthur of the Sixth Royal Veteran Battalion. In 1838, Ballow was appointed assistant colonial surgeon and the young couple moved to Brisbane where the doctor took charge of Her Majesty's General Hospital, Moreton Bay, towards the end of the convict era. The number of convicts had dwindled to about three hundred from a maximum of approximately a thousand in 1831. In 1839, the government decided to close the penal settlement altogether, but it was not until 1842 that Moreton Bay was thrown open for free settlement. This did not mean that Ballow's services were no longer required officially. A detachment of military, some prisoners and government officials still remained. However, even before 1842, people other than convicts and their keepers were coming to the settlement. At first, there were no medical facilities for them. In

1841, Ballow pointed out to Lieutenant Gorman, the commandant, that there were many who could not officially be treated and he sought permission to borrow medicines from the hospital dispensary, promising to replace them from stock he had ordered from Sydney. Having Gorman's approval, he thus became the first hospital superintendent with the right of private practice in what was later to become Queensland.

From well preserved documents in the Queensland State Archives, it can be seen that Ballow was a sound practitioner. His clinical notes were well-kept and he took an interest in the efficacy of his treatment. In 1845 he wrote to his superior in Sydney, giving an account of his observations over a period of several months of the results of potassium iodide treatment. Ballow claimed that the drug was a highly useful remedial agent which could be used with the greatest safety in rheumatism, glandular conditions and the after-effects of syphilis. It improved the appetite, was a powerful tonic, and patients looked more cheerful and clearer in complexion as a result. Of course some treatments, acceptable at the time, would be frowned on today. When a John McCallum was admitted to the hospital with "much bruising about the feet and legs in being washed ashore after the *Sovereign* was wrecked at Amity Point" in 1847, Ballow considered that he should be bled. Twenty ounces of blood were taken in hospital, in addition to that he had lost in battling the waves. In those days leeches were applied for black eyes and amputations were effected without anaesthetic. When that energetic advocate of migration, Rev. John Dunmore Lang, asked for an opinion of the effect of Moreton Bay settlement's climate on health, the Scottish doctor replied:

> The district of Moreton Bay is altogether an extremely healthy one, very few deaths occurring from disease of any kind. Intermittent fever prevails in certain localities, more particularly in the neighbourhood of swampy grounds, and in situations where there is no free current of air to drive off the miasmata arising from decaying vegetable matter. This malady occurs at times only, chiefly after long continued rains and most cases is mild in its attacks, soon yields to treatment, leaves no permanent bad effects and has never to my knowledge been fatal. Rheumatic affections are probably more frequent than any other form of disease; but these also, at least, in my experience, soon give way under a use of remedies and subsequent attacks may be guarded against by a moderate degree of precaution.
>
> Diseases of the liver and of the stomach and bowels, are, I think considering the latitudes (27°–30°), by no means frequent and in those

areas where the first named viscus is affected there is generally merely functional derangements — organic disease being rarely met with.

Women generally get over their confinements easily, puerperal or childbed fever being seldom seen; indeed, I recollect but one case only during my eight years practice here and in that case the woman had been ailing for some time previous to delivery.

Children thrive well and all the ailments and diseases incident to infancy and childhood are mild in their attacks and soon got over.

I think the best character I can give the climate is to say of it that it is by no means a profitable field for practitioners of medicine.

Ballow's original book of accounts contains the names of many notables in early Brisbane society. Ten visits to the Petries between 1846 and 1849 were settled by contract. Captain Wickham, the police magistrate in charge of the settlement, and his family were his private patients. The records show that Ballow called in Kearsey Cannan, for a time his only medical colleague in Brisbane, for consultation at Mrs Wickham's confinement. It is interesting to note that the doctor handed twenty-seven accounts to a debt-collector named Power and that gentleman succeeded in having twenty-one paid.

The government decided to close the convict hospital early in 1848. Ballow was given an opportunity to transfer as assistant colonial surgeon in Van Diemen's Land. When he refused the offer he left the colonial medical service. When a civilian committee opened the hospital again for public use in 1849, the Scot was appointed house surgeon. When no longer employed by the government as colonial surgeon, he was offered official positions outside the field of medicine. He was both a coroner and a magistrate.

In the two years following his appointment as a coroner, Ballow conducted no fewer than twenty-eight enquiries into deaths in the settlement, outside Brisbane. At the time it was the practice for a jury to assist the coroner. A newspaper report tells how Ballow and a jury of five travelled on horseback from Brisbane to the Bush Inn below Cunningham's Gap when a man died in a dray accident. On another occasion his jury accompanied him to Flinders Peak twenty miles from Ipswich to examine the exhumed body of Joshua Crow, who was murdered on a sheep station there. The following extract from the *Moreton Bay Courier* reveals the rather irregular conduct of this enquiry, in which Ballow acted both as coroner and medical witness.

During the inquest held on the deceased, Joshua Crow, the surgeon,

> Mr. Wilks who had made a post mortem examination of the body, the result of which he had written down and deposed to, being absent on professional business, the jury had not the advantage of examining him as to the probable means by which the wounds on the body had been inflicted. To supply this deficiency the coroner, in his medical capacity, gave evidence on that point to the jury. This is one of the contingencies anticipated, both in England and this colony and which was advanced as a reason why the office should always be held by a professional gentleman.

Although Edward Wilks had been sent by Dr McTaggart Dorsey, an Ipswich magistrate, to conduct the post-mortem, he was not on the register of medical practitioners held by the New South Wales medical board. This was not an uncommon occurrence in those early days, but Ballow saw fit to report the fact to the attorney general in Sydney. Of Ballow's twenty-eight cases, he found that six deaths had been deliberately caused by another person; nine had been accidental — five of these by drowning; and three were due to natural causes, although one death had been accelerated by drinking. In seven deaths the coroner gave as his finding: "Visitation by God".

In his capacity as a magistrate, however, Dr Ballow was involved in an incident which brought him some temporary discredit. It started with a man called Henry Humby, who lived with his family in a hut at York's Hollow (now Victoria Park) on the outskirts of Brisbane. Around dusk one evening in November 1849, a young Aborigine told Humby that members of his tribe nearby had hamstrung one of John Petrie's bullocks ready for roasting, and had designs on others. Humby, who the *Moreton Bay Courier* said "had in his composition an unusual proportion of the elements of folly and cowardice", became terrified and locked himself in his hut, giving "full scope to his fancy and conjuring up through the darkness a host of imaginary hostile natives". After two hours of worrying he crept away with his wife, leaving their children in the hut with a dog. The couple hastened into Brisbane to tell Petrie what they believed was happening to his bullocks and what they feared was about to happen to the town at the hands of Aborigines on the warpath. Petrie, who was on friendly terms with the Aborigines and who had missed some bullocks, went to the camp to investigate. On arrival, he found no sign of any fire and persuaded two of the Aborigines to help him to look for his bullocks.

Meanwhile, Humby and his wife ran to the house of Chief Constable John Fitzpatrick with an even more embellished tale.

Fitzpatrick, who was in bed, detailed a constable to inform the nearest magistrate and then went back to bed. Captain Wickham, the police magistrate, lived at Newstead House three miles from the centre of the town. Ballow, as the nearest magistrate, received the frightened Humby's story of Aborigines preparing to attack the town. The doctor did not know how to handle the matter. After conferring with Lieutenant Cameron, the officer of the military detachment in the settlement, he directed him to handle the problem as he saw fit. Cameron decided to take his men to the camp but Ballow declined to accompany him. As the troops neared the camp they divided into two groups with the idea of surrounding the natives. A report of the incident states that a boomerang was thrown at one group and the soldiers replied with rifle fire, wounding four of the natives. There is some confusion on this point and it is arguable whether the boomerang could have been seen in the dark. A quarter of a mile away Petrie heard the shots and returned to the camp. He explained to Lieutenant Cameron that the Aborigines had no hostile intentions and Cameron led his soldiers back to their barracks.

When Governor Fitzroy received the report of the incident, he was very critical of the conduct of the Moreton Bay officials. Chief Constable Fitzpatrick was dismissed for returning to bed after Humby's terrified warning and not investigating the story. Lieutenant Cameron and Ballow received letters of censure, and Ballow was told that his conduct in directing Lieutenant Cameron to call out his detachment, and then not going with them, appeared to have been inexcusable and deserving severe censure. Ballow's error of judgment does not appear to have altered his standing in the community. In the same mail as the letter of censure came the advice that he had been appointed surgeon to the gaol, and in addition to his medical work he continued as magistrate and coroner.

In mid-August 1850, Wickham received information that the ship *Emigrant*, carrying migrants for the settlement, had arrived in Moreton Bay with sickness aboard. As there was no permanent appointment of health officer at the settlement, he asked Ballow to act in this capacity and inspect the ship.

The *Emigrant*, classed A.1 at Lloyd's, was owned by John de Wolfe and on his behalf had been tendered by brokers to the emigration commissioners for the conveyance of migrants from Plymouth in England to Moreton Bay, at the rate of £11.9s.0d for each adult passenger. She had been built at St John, New Brunswich, in 1845, a vessel 140 feet long, of 680 tons under the old measurement, and 753 by the new measurement of the day. She left Plymouth under the command of Captain William Kemp with George Mitchell as surgeon superintendent on April 17. One document gives a figure of 235 adult migrants, whilst another report states that 261 arrived alive in Moreton Bay. No matter which of these two totals is correct, it may be safely assumed that the migrants — English and Irish with a few from Scotland — were crowded on the small ship. After leaving Plymouth, the vessel's course was the usual one taken at that time from England to Australia. She sailed down the west coast of Africa and then around the Cape of Good Hope to catch the roaring forties to Australia. The ship's surgeon, Mitchell, told Ballow that while the ship was in the vicinity of Cape Verde on the west coast of Africa, typhus fever made its appearance among the migrants. From that time till the *Emigrant* arrived in Moreton Bay eighteen died aboard the vessel, fourteen from typhus and four from other causes.

Typhus fever was once the most important disease in the world's history. The responsible organism is spread from person to person by the human body louse and enters the body when louse faeces are rubbed into abrasions during scratching. As the various names for the disease suggest — camp fever, gaol fever, famine fever and ship fever — it often occurs where there is overcrowding. It is credited with having decided wars in the middle ages: armies decimated by the fever were unable to fight. In severe cases the early symptoms of fever — headache, pain in the back and limbs with a rash — are followed by prostration, mental lethargy, heart weakness and muttering delirium. Death comes from exhaustion and heart failure. Before the advent of antibiotics there was no specific treatment.

Ballow ordered the ship to proceed to a position off Dunwich on Stradbroke Island, which, only a few months before, had been proclaimed as a quarantine station but which had as yet no facilities. Wickham then engaged the ketch *Aurora* as a means of communication between the quarantine station and Brisbane, and proceeded down the bay, taking Goerge Watson, the emigration agent, to act as superintendent of quarantine, and four "pensioners" — ticket of leave convicts who had arrived not long before on the *Bangalore* — to act as guards. At Dunwich Wickham formally ordered the ship, crew and passengers into quarantine.

The tragic hardships of the voyage from England were to continue for another three months on Stradbroke Island. The dilapidated buildings at Dunwich which had once formed a convict outpost provided no shelter. Wickham supplied twelve small tents and the ship sent sails and awnings ashore for living quarters and a hospital in which to nurse those suffering from the fever. Dr Patrick Mallon, who had recently come to Moreton Bay, volunteered to take medical charge of the quarantine station. The ship's doctor, George Mitchell, could offer no help to Mallon. Shortly after the ship's arrival he developed early symptoms of the disease and died a month later. Poor Mitchell, realizing that he would not recover, gave written directions for the disposal of the gratuity due to him for his services on the voyage. His letter is preserved in the Mitchell Library, Sydney. Part of the letter read:

> To the owners of ship as per order given to Capt. Kemp, the sum of thirty pounds. The remainder to be forwarded to my mother (if alive), Mrs Jane Mitchell, relict of the late Alex Mitchell, Cladybeg, Mucket Hill, County Armagh, Ireland and if my mother not alive to be divided amongst my sisters.

The graves of Ballow and Mitchell at Dunwich, Stradbroke Island. The two doctors died fighting typhus fever brought to Moreton Bay in the ship *Emigrant*.

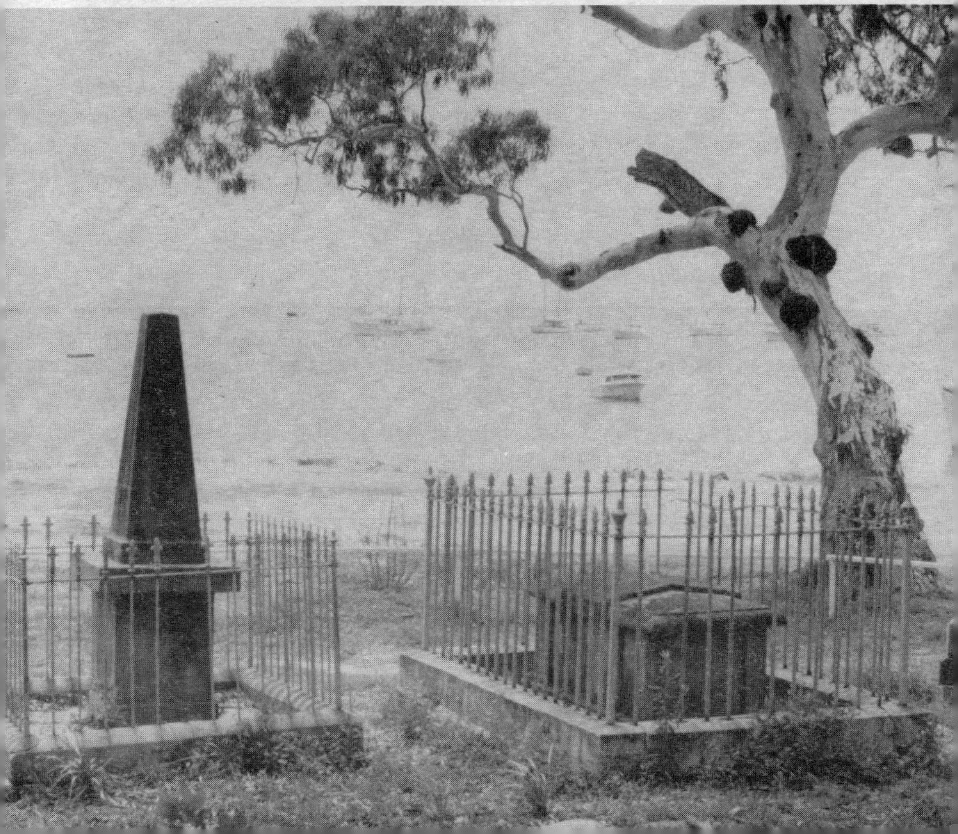

Mitchell was due to receive £130.10s.0d calculated on the basis of ten shillings for each migrant who arrived alive at Moreton Bay. It was not long before Mallon also developed the disease. Wickham approached the doctors at Brisbane and Ipswich for relief for Mallon. Of the six available only Ballow offered his services. This refusal by the medical practitioners to volunteer was not frowned on by the community. The *Moreton Bay Courier* regarded the refusals as "natural and not at all surprising" and went on to say:

> The want of zeal (on the part of the doctors) may be traced to the fact, that there is no certain provision for the surviving families of those who may be cut off by disease in the performance of such dangerous duties, and although we should join in admiration of any man who would voluntarily risk his life for the preservation of others, it must be remembered that there are grave and solemn duties which every man owes to those dependent upon him for support, and which must be allowed to have their full weight in the consideration of this question. If the only thing to be considered was, whether a professional man should place his life in jeopardy for the purposes of arresting the ravages of a fatal disorder, or shelter himself under the plea of danger, we conceive that the former course would be pronounced the course of duty; but that is not the only consideration when such professional men have wives, children, or other helpless relatives in their care. In such case, it would undoubtedly be a duty, and a very serious one, to calculate the risk of such dependants being left destitute by the death of their protector, and if such a probability was made manifest, it would he hard to condemn any man who gave his first care to his family. Whilst we appreciate and honour the devotion of those who have exposed themselves to death in the performance of their professional duties, we cannot say that he who has no prospect of his family being provided for, ought to be blamed for being careful of his life.
>
> The cause of such scruples is plainly the neglect of the Government and Legislature to provide a fund for compensating the widows and orphans of medical men who die in attending to such cases of public calamity as those which have recently occurred in our harbour. If the family of the soldier who loses his life in destroying human life be thought worthy of provision, surely he whose mission it is to preserve life should not be left without a similar incentive to action. As far as the profession of medicine is superior in humanity and usefulness to that of arms, so far we consider that the claim of compensation for the family of a medical man who should die in the public service would be superior to such a claim on the part of the survivors of a soldier or a sailor who perished in battle.

Volunteering, Ballow pointed out that he was not obliged to do so as he no longer held the official appointment of colonial surgeon.

He went on to say that in addition to the risk of infection he was making a very considerable sacrifice regarding his private practice, and that as there was no proper accommodation to afford shelter at Dunwich from the inclemencies of the weather and as there was a vast amount of sickness, the duty was very arduous and disagreeable. The risk to Ballow was indeed real. After spending five weeks on the island he, too, developed typhus and died. Fortunately, Mallon had recovered and was able to continue to care for the patients still contracting the disease. Apart from Dr Ballow and Dr Mitchell, the fever claimed twenty-five victims from the passengers and crew. Two other tragic deaths occurred at the quarantine station. A young woman who could not stand the strain committed suicide by drowning, and a boy died after falling into a fire whilst his parents were attending Ballow's funeral service. Slowly the epidemic ran its course, but it was not until November, more than three months from the date that the *Emigrant* arrived in Moreton Bay, that the survivors came up the river to Brisbane. The fever accounted for over forty deaths.

When Wickham's report of the arrival of the ship with illness aboard reached Sydney he was asked by the immigration agent to conduct an enquiry to determine whether or not the blame for the epidemic could be laid at anyone's door. He enlisted the services of William Duncan, sub-collector of customs at Moreton Bay, to sit on a board of immigration with him. Dr Kearsey Cannan, now acting as health officer, gave the board medical advice. Both Wickham and Cannan made several trips to the quarantine station, both during the enquiry and later, but neither took any part in the immediate management at Dunwich. The board's report praised the efforts of the ship's master, Captain Kemp, and the surgeon superintendent, Mitchell. It said that "Captain Kemp is deserving of the very highest commendation. The migrants are unanimous in testifying to his humane and indefatigable exertions to mitigate the fearful calamity which their voyage attended. The conduct of the late surgeon superintendent, Dr Mitchell was under the most trying circumstances in every respect praiseworthy." The only suggestion made as to the cause of the disaster was that it could have arisen from the fact that on a previous voyage the vessel had carried guano — seabird droppings collected as manure — and some of this substance remaining on board had fermented. In the days when the true nature of epidemics was not yet known this was not an unreasonable submission. The *Moreton Bay Courier* paid tribute to another who rendered great service to the sick on the passage out:

> But there was one on board upon whom no official responsibility devolved, and who was yet, to use the language of Scott, "a ministering angel" to the sick. Mrs Kemp, the Captain's wife, has indeed earned golden opinions from all sorts of people. This lady, as appears by the statements of all the witnesses examined, was unremitting in her charitable attentions to the passengers, and even when suffering from fatigue and exhaustion, devoted herself with a singular and rare humanity to the alleviation of the sorrows and sufferings of others.

Ballow's wife, who received a gratuity of £300 from the government, erected a tombstone over her husband's grave at Dunwich. The inscription reads:

> To The Memory Of
> DAVID KEITH BALLOW
> LATE COLONIAL SURGEON, CORONER OF THE DISTRICT, AND MAGISTRATE OF THE TERRITORY: WHO IN THE DISCHARGE OF HIS DUTY AS SURGEON SUPERINTENDENT OF THE QUARANTINE STATION
> Fell with many others, whose graves lie around
> A victim of Typhus Fever
> Born at Montrose, October 27th 1804, Died September 29th 1850
> "Greater love hath no man than this that a man lay down his life for friends" 15th Chap. St John 13th Verse.
> This tomb was erected by his affectionate widow
> MARGARET CAMPBELL BALLOW

Similar inscriptions may be read on plaques in St John's Cathedral, Ann Street, and on the facade of Ballow Chambers, Wickham Terrace, Brisbane, named in his honour.

Moreton Bay's First Anaesthetist

> The thought of an operation was torture and patients suffered agonies beforehand; finally tied to the table and held by force, they tore madly at their straps, shrieking in uncontrolled terror — the one saving aspect of the whole ghastly affair was that no one understood the meaning of surgical shock. The soporific draughts of Dioscorides and the sleeping sponges of the Middle Ages were forgotten or discarded as unreliable. Haste was the great thing and he was the best surgeon who operated fastest. Robert Liston amputed the thigh by compressing the artery with his left hand and cutting and sawing with his right. If he needed the use of both hands he held the saw between his teeth. Liston's knife flashed and if the spectator sneezed or winked or turned his head he missed the operation because it was over. In spite of his speed Liston had harrowing memories; a man who was to be cut for stone lost his courage on the operating table, rushed down the long corridor and locked himself in the lavatory until Liston made a battering-ram of his powerful shoulder, broke the door and carried the patient back.

The above account from Victor Robinson's history of medicine rather graphically describes surgery before anaesthetic was discovered in America in the 1840s. The soporific draught Robinson referred to was Mandrake wine, used in surgical operations by Nero's army surgeon, Dioscorides. The sleeping sponges of the Middle Ages were saturated with opium, hyoscyamus, mandragora, conium and other narcotics and held over the patient's nose. Convicts and their keepers, who were the first white inhabitants of Moreton Bay, and the free settlers who came before the use of anaesthetics, would have suffered similar torture under the surgeon's knife. In some cases their agonies would have been lessened by rum intoxication, which many surgeons regarded as an appropriate pre-operative medication.

For some years before their value as anaesthetics was recognized, laughing gas (nitrous oxide) and ether were used as amusements at parties and ether frolics. They were first used to deaden the pain of operations during dental extractions. An American dentist, Wells, decided to demonstrate the value of laughing gas as an anaesthetic to a surgeon named Warren and several medical students. However, the patient did not receive enough anaesthetic and cried out when the tooth was extracted, whereupon the medical students shouted "Humbug". Then another dentist, Morton, persuaded Warren to let him use ether while a tumour was removed from a young woman's neck. The patient made no movement or sound during the operation. This time, Dr Warren turned to his audience and said, "Gentlemen, this is no humbug". The day was 16 October 1846. The next year James Young Simpson, professor of Obstetrics at Glasgow University, used another agent, chloroform, to relieve the pain of childbirth.

There is some dispute as to who was the first to use anaesthetics in Australia. William Russ Pugh, a Launceston surgeon, and John Belisario, a Sydney dentist, vie for the honour. Press reports of the administration of ether by the two appeared about the same time in June 1847. Pugh is credited with removing a tumour from a girl's jaw and a cataract from a man's eye after ether had been administered. Belisario announced in the *Sydney Morning Herald* of 15 June 1847 that he was "enabled by means of the recent discovery, ether inhalation, to perform the most difficult operations in dental surgery, with perfect freedom from pain or subsequent inconvenience to his patients". He was supported by a statement from Charles Nathan, surgeon, who declared that the inhalation of ether was harmless. Some Sydney surgeons also began using the two agents. However, not all in the medical profession were enchanted with the use of the new agents. The editor of the *Australian Medical Journal* in June 1847 wrote the following rather sceptical comments:

> For minor operations in surgery we would consider any such measures as unnecessary; in the more important ones we think it will be found not infrequently conducive to secondary consequences of a grave character, even if it did not in many constitutions produce effects of a mischievous nature. We have no hesitation in predicting for this process a transient popularity; it will have its day, ultimately to be abandoned as useless and, or injurious.

Credit for the administration of the first anaesthetic in Moreton Bay has for many years been given to William Hobbs, who used chloroform while Hugh Bell removed a cancer from the testis of a Chinese named Chong in 1854. Hobbs had arrived at Moreton Bay in 1849 as surgeon on the *Chaseley*, one of John Dunmore Lang's immigrant ships. The migrants were impressed with Hobbs's services during the voyage and, as was the custom, told him so in a letter published in the *Moreton Bay Courier* of 19 May 1849:

TO WILLIAM HOBBS, ESQ.,
Surgeon Superintendent of the Chaseley

We, the undersigned passengers per Chaseley, beg to return you our warmest thanks for your uniform kindness and attention during the passage to this colony. Of the natural goodness of your heart there cannot be two opinions; and we hope that if it should be our lot and yours to remain in this district, a reciprocity of those good feelings may be maintained, which were commenced under such favourable auspices.

With every desire for your welfare and happiness we have the honour to remain,

Your obedient servants,

[The original document contained the signatures of more than seventy passengers.]

After putting up his plate for a few months at Drayton, Toowoomba, Hobbs returned to Brisbane where he served as visiting surgeon to the Brisbane Hospital, as government health officer, and in many other positions for many years. Hugh Bell came to Brisbane as surgeon superintendent on the *Parsee* after graduating from Guy's Hospital, London. He became house surgeon at the Brisbane Hospital and later built up a large private practice.

The register of cases and treatment contains the description of the operation on the Chinese man to whom Hobbs gave chloroform. (The register is kept in the Queensland State Archives.) The notes on the surgery performed include a reference to the deftness with which surgeon Bell carried the incision round behind the testicle with a sweep. Progress notes on the case state that Chong "got well without a bad symptom and was discharged cured". These optimistic remarks were rather misplaced, for the patient returned in a few months for more surgery. The *Moreton Bay Courier* was so impressed with the first operation on Chong that it published the following account a few days after it was performed.

Successful Operation in the Brisbane Hospital. — An operation of considerable interest has lately been performed by Dr Bell, House Surgeon in the Brisbane Hospital, upon Chong, a Chinaman, for the removal of a large ulcerating cancerous tumour, fourteen inches in circumference, from the lower part of the abdomen. Chloroform was successfully, and in this case advantageously, administered by Dr Hobbs, the operation requiring much careful dissection, as it was necessary to pass into the abdomen and expose the intestines in order to pass a ligature above the neck of the tumour. On recovery from the effects of the chloroform, the patient stated that he was conscious of the opera-

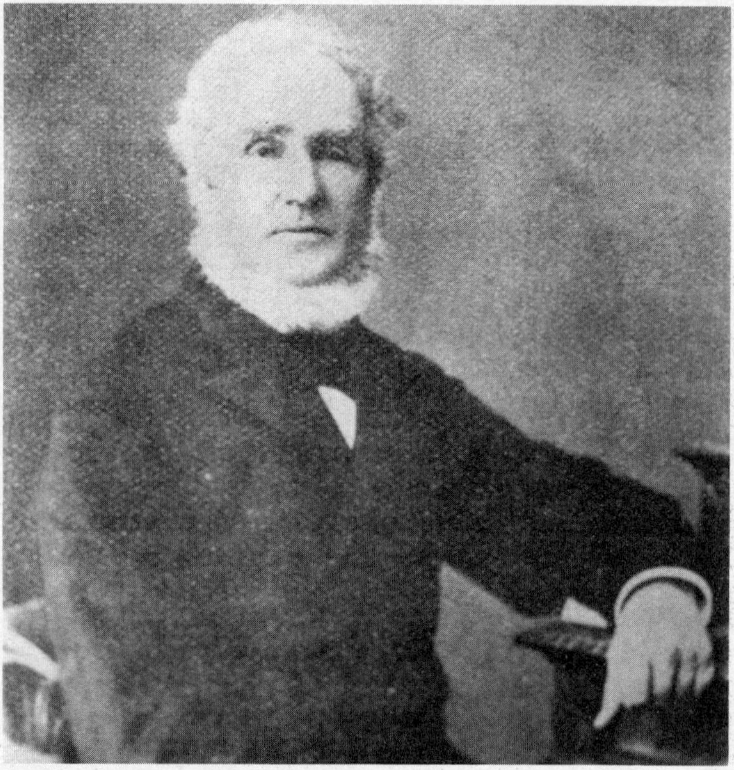

William Hobbs, around 1885, one of Moreton Bay's first anaesthetists. (Courtesy Commonwealth Department of Health)

> tion. It had not been deemed advisable to continue complete insensibility during the operation which occupied nearly half an hour. The disease was of so serious a nature that it was much doubted — even if the patient did not die under the operation which was by no means impossible — whether he would be radically cured or not. The excruciating pain he suffered, and the apparent improbability of his surviving more than a few weeks, as the case stood, were the inducements to operate with so little chance of ultimate recovery. The patient was admitted on the 27th June; operated on the 10th July; had less pain immediately after the operation than for weeks before; recovered without a bad symptom and discharged, quite cured, on the 7th August. It was with difficulty that he was confined to hospital during the last week. We record this case as one out of very many showing the great benefits derivable from the Brisbane Hospital.

Two pertinent facts emerge from this report. The article states that chloroform was administered *in this case advantageously.*

These words suggest that there had been previous cases in which anaesthetic had been given disadvantageously. The date of the operation was July 1854 — seven years after the first anaesthetic was given in Australia. The question arises as to whether the doctors at Moreton Bay were conservative and had heeded the prediction of the editor of the *Australian Medical Journal* that the new procedure would be abandoned as useless and/or injurious. Had they really waited seven years to administer the first anaesthetic? Or had researchers missed reports of earlier use of chloroform and ether? These points prompted further research. I studied the Brisbane Hospital records again and combed the files of the *Moreton Bay Courier* for relevant articles. The results showed that while the Brisbane medicos were not as quick as their southern colleagues to adopt the use of anaesthetics, they had recognized their value some years before Hobbs had asked Chong to inhale chloroform.

The following points in the story came to light. It is true that the Brisbane Hospital records contain no earlier reference to the administration of ether or chloroform than the oft-quoted case of Bell's operation on Chong. However, there is a gap in the records of over two years from 26 October 1850 to 8 January 1853. A register of cases and treatment for this period did not reach the archives. The *Moreton Bay Courier* contains references to anaesthetics for this period and there are some interesting points worth noting in the issues for the years before this. In the 5 August 1848 edition, J. Taggart, a pharmacist of Queen Street, advertised chloroform for sale. The agent was available to all and sundry, for there were no poisons regulations to prevent any man purchasing the drug if he so wished. But when the Brisbane Hospital asked druggists to quote prices for the supply of drugs for 1849, chloroform was not in the list of items required. The hospital asked suppliers to quote for ether by the ounce. Such small quantities of ether, and the absence of chloroform from the drugs supply list suggests that not many, if any, anaesthetics were contemplated. In November 1849, the following article appeared in the *Moreton Bay Courier*:

> Surgery In The Bush. — A correspondent at Drayton communicates the following: On Saturday last a man named Brewer, in the employment of Mr Wiggins fell from the top of a dray-load of wool, on its way through this place to Ipswich, the wheel passing over the right hand, arm and fleshy part of the thigh. Fortunately, Dr Mallon was here, who pronounced that an amputation of the limb was necessary. This gentleman having been some days previously called from Brisbane to

> attend another patient, was unprovided with instruments: but — "Necessitas habet legem" — he substituted a common knife and saw and leathern strap. Matters thus arranged, with no better assistance than that of a bullock-driver, the limb was speedily amputated and the man is now rapidly recovering.

As Dr Mallon had none of his instruments with him, he probably had no anaesthetic agent either and it is presumed the operation was performed without it. In 1849 and 1850 there are records of three amputations but no reference to anaesthetic being used. The Brisbane Hospital register contains a rather terse account by David Ballow, house surgeon, when he examined Joseph Willis, whose leg was crushed when a tree fell on him. Ballow wrote in the register: "Immediate amputation necessary, which was accordingly performed".

Then, on 14 June 1851, the *Moreton Bay Courier* carried this article:

> CHLOROFORM. — The value of this agent in alleviating pain to mankind is becoming generally acknowledged throughout this colony. A few days ago an instance occurred in Brisbane, in which its peculiar properties were used during the performance of what otherwise would have been a painful operation. A man, named Peardon, in the employment, we believe, of Mr Hodgson, came to the Brisbane Hospital with a bad thumb, occasioned by a neglected whitlow, and Dr Swift, the officer under whose charge the patient was placed, directed that the thumb should be amputated. This operation was accordingly performed by Dr Barton the House Surgeon, in the presence of Dr Swift, the patient having previously inhaled chloroform. He informed us two days afterwards that he had not felt the slightest pain, and the wound was then healthy. He has since been discharged, cured.

And so it appears that William Hobbs was not the first anaesthetist, as has been believed. The honour must go to Dr Jacob Meade Swift, presuming it was he who asked his patient to inhale chloroform before surgeon Barton amputated the thumb.

Love and Blindness

In the twenty years before Moreton Bay settlement became a separate colony at the end of 1859, pioneers pushed out from Brisbane and the Darling Downs, which had been settled by the Leslie brothers in 1840. As the pastoralists settled, small towns grew up, and medical practitioners put up their plates signifying their willingness to tend the ill. The facilities were primitive. For a number of years the only public hospital was in Brisbane — generally too far away to allow easy transfer of patients. Some early doctors established small hospitals, often no more than slab huts, to care for those who could not be nursed in their homes. William Dorsey, the first active private medical practitioner in Moreton Bay, opened a hospital at Little Ipswich but when practicable, he transferred the severe cases to Brisbane by bullock dray or boat. An early doctor on the Darling Downs, William Miles, admitted the sick and injured to his hospital at Ryford, near Clifton, and Hart Brown conducted a similar institution at Gayndah. These were private hospitals — if they could be flattered by such an appellation.

The first public hospital outside Brisbane was established in Maryborough. In a letter dated Saturday afternoon, 17 May 1856, Dr Edward Fielding Palmer wrote to the colonial secretary advising that a hospital committee had been formed in Maryborough. He requested a subsidy of £200 to add to a similar sum that he expected to be raised locally to build and equip a hospital. The hospital began functioning in March 1859 in a slab-construction building lined with calico.

At that time, the men who practised medicine in the Moreton Bay settlement fell into three groups. First came a group who were registered with the New South Wales medical board. A second group comprised practitioners who were well-trained but whose names were not on the register. Some of these had not even bothered to apply for registration. Some had degrees from the continent of Europe and elsewhere which the medical board did not recognize. Thirdly, scattered throughout the country, were men with varying degrees of medical knowledge to whom the pioneers often turned gladly when no one else was available.

Edward Fielding Palmer, a leader in establishing the Maryborough Hospital, was one of the registered practitioners. Also in Maryborough at the time was Gustav Ernst, who held a degree from a medical school in Germany which the medical board did not recognize. The lack of registration did not bother the Maryborough Hospital committee: it was satisfied with Ernst's reputation as a doctor and appointed him visiting surgeon to the hospital.

In February 1860, Emily DeCaux, aged sixteen, was admitted to the hospital with incipient blindness. About a week later, when she was the only patient in the women's ward, Dr Ernst entered, unattended. After enquiring about her eyes, there was silence. Then, according to evidence the girl gave later, he placed his hands under the bed clothes and on her person. He took the girl's hand and placed it on his person. When she remonstrated, the doctor told her not to be foolish and that that was what she wanted. He said also that if she slept with him one night she would "have her eyes right" in the morning. On another occasion, he threw himself upon her at full length. The girl complained to the matron but no action was taken. However, when a visitor told the patient a few days later that accounts of the incidents with Ernst were common gossip in the town, it was decided to report the offence to the police. A charge of indecent assault was laid against Ernst and he appeared before a magistrate. The *Moreton Bay Courier* reported the hearing:

> The case was heard in open court and frightful were the details. The doctor offered her tarts and cakes, telling her she would have her sight again by his sleeping with her. The matron was informed by the unfortunate child, who did not report, believing, as she said, "that no harm had been done". A searching investigation and the correction of many great irregularities which have hitherto been perpetrated with impunity in this place, is much needed.

Ernst was committed to stand trial at the next Maryborough assizes and was allowed bail. He had to wait for nearly ten months before he appeared before Mr Justice Lutwyche and a jury of twelve. In his summing up Judge Lutwyche said it was remarkable that no character witness had been called by the defendant's counsel, but that might be explained by the fact that the defendant was so well-known as to make that course unnecessary. He must be presumed, therefore, to bear a good character. Likewise, there had been nothing added to injure the character of the young woman. After a brief retirement the jury returned a verdict of guilty, with a strong recommendation to mercy. Addressing the prisoner, Judge Lutwyche said:

> Gustav Ernst, you have been found guilty of two charges of indecent assault. In the first instance a recommendation to mercy was made by the jury. To these recommendations I have always paid the greatest attention, consistent with my duty. Your offences are of a very aggravated kind. Under ordinary circumstances they might not have been considered very serious; but as a medical man your profession gives you an entrance into every family — and this, with your position as the medical officer of a public institution makes these most grievous charges. I trust the punishment you will soon undergo will have a marked influence on your future career wherever you may go, for your reputation will not allow your remaining in these colonies. I sentence you to two years imprisonment with hard labour for each offence, the two sentences to be concurrent.

Ernst was taken to Brisbane Gaol to serve the sentence, the maximum the law provided for the offence. Judge Lutwyche's opinion that the doctor's reputation would be so tarnished that he would leave the colony proved to be quite erroneous. Less than six months after he was convicted, the citizens of Maryborough and Musket Flat, a small settlement twenty-five miles away, had other beliefs. Both groups sent petitions to Governor Bowen for the mitigation of the sentence. The petition from Maryborough read:

> His Excellency,
> Sir George Ferguson Bowen,
> Governor of Queensland and the Honourable Executive Council,
> We, the undersigned inhabitants of Maryborough and the Wide Bay district most respectfully beg you will take into your merciful considerations the case of Gustav Ernst, M.D. who was sentenced to two years imprisonment at the last March Assizes holden at Maryborough for an assault upon one Emily DeCaux.
>
> Your petitioners beg to state they always had the greatest confidence in Dr Ernst as medical man and very much deplore the loss of his services, as up to the time he was found guilty of the offence charged with he bore an excellent character while staying with your petitioners for 3 years upwards.
>
> Your petitioners beg to remind your Honourable Council that Dr Ernst was held to bail for nearly 12 months previous to his trial consequently in itself a severe punishment to a person of his profession — many of your petitioners would gladly have given testimony at the trial as to the previous good character of Dr Ernst but in consequence of some unaccountable misunderstanding were not called upon to do so.

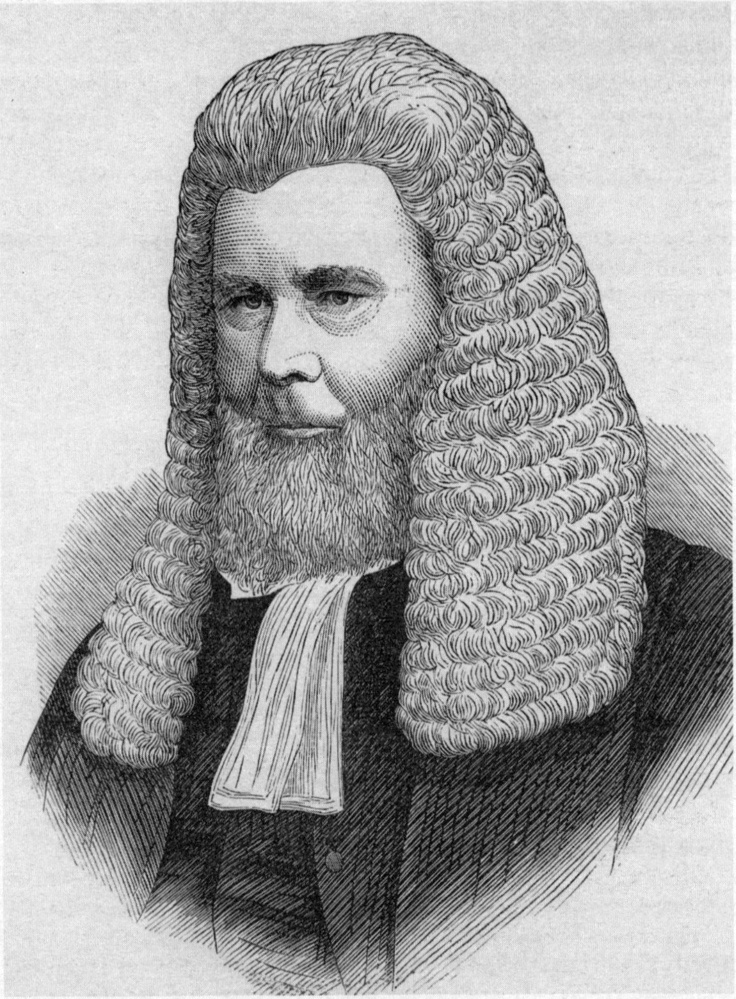

Judge Lutwyche (around 1875), who sentenced Dr Ernst to two years' imprisonment. (Courtesy Oxley Library)

Your petitioners sincerely hope you will take a merciful view of the case as they are anxious to restore the prisoner again to society, this being the first appeal for mercy that ever emanated from the inhabitants of Wide Bay to Your Excellency's most Honourable Council, they respectfully trust that Your Excellency will take a favourable and considerate view of this case now before Your Excellency and that you will grant the request of the Inhabitants of Wide Bay, who in duty bound will Ever Pray.

Ninety-four signatures were attached to the petition. The first three were those of Emily Decaux, the blind girl herself, her mother, Mary White, and her stepfather, Elijah White. These three signatures were in the same handwriting. The next to sign were the twelve jurors at the hearing, followed by the citizens of Maryborough and district. The citizens of Musket Flat came straight to the point. They were without the services of their doctor and wanted him back. They said they deeply regretted his loss and trusted that His Excellency would take the matter into consideration and restore him to the district from which he was taken. When the petition was received in Brisbane, it was referred to Judge Lutwyche for comments. His reply included the following:

> In passing sentence, I expressed my regret that I could not attend to the recommendation of mercy made by the jury, as I was of opinion that an offence of an unusually grave character had been committed. The conduct of the defendant led me to the conclusion that he had formed a deliberate design to inflame the girl's passions, and afterwards debauch her person, and I told the jury that conduct of this kind was greatly aggravated by the circumstance that the girl was blind, and that the defendant was not only a medical man, in whom families are obliged to repose a great amount of confidence, but the medical officer of a public institution. I accordingly passed upon him the heaviest sentence which the law awards for offences of this description.
>
> I observe with some surprise and more pain that the only reason assigned in one of the petitions (from Musket Flat) for the release of Dr Ernst from prison is that the petitioners regret the loss of Dr Ernst's medical services in the district. It does not appear to have occurred to any one of the persons who signed that petition that the salutory result of a great example might reasonably be looked upon as outweighing the personal inconvenience occasioned by the absence of a particular medical practitioner in the district from which the petition proceeded.
>
> The other petition from Maryborough, alleges that Dr Ernst bore an excellent character for three years before he was convicted of the offence, and states that many of the petitioners (not, however, specifying their names) would gladly have borne testimony to that effect at the trial, but that in consequence of some unaccountable misunderstanding they were not called upon to do so. I am not prepared to say that such evidence would not have had some weight with me in apportioning punishment, if the evidence had been given at the proper time, and had stood the test of a cross-examination by the Attorney General. As the case stood, however there was nothing to induce me to pass a lighter sentence than the defendant received, and,

after the trial, information reached me that if evidence as to character had been tendered, it would have still further damaged the defendant's reputation. A gentleman of high standing in the town called on me before I left Maryborough on the part of himself and others, who, while acknowledging the justice of the sentence, were anxious for a remission of the "hard labour" portion of it. In the course of conversation I expressed some astonishment that in a place where Dr Ernst had been so long known, no one had come forward to give him a character. Whereupon I was told that it would have been useless — that his character where women were concerned would not bear investigation in a Court of Justice. I believe, therefore, that there was no "misunderstanding" on the subject, and that the defendant's counsel exercised a wise discretion by not calling witnesses to character.

In conclusion, I may observe, that it has come to my knowledge that great efforts were made before the trial to keep the principal witness out of the way, so that she might not give evidence against Dr Ernst. After the trial her stepfather, whose name is annexed to the petition, and who has signed it for her and her mother (with what authority does not appear) refused to receive her in his house or to contribute anything towards her support, and but for the assistance of some persons, who raised a small sum of money, and sent her down to the Brisbane Hospital, she must have starved. Under all the circumstances I have no hesitation in saying that it is impossible for me to support the prayer of the petitions, or even to recommend any mitigation of Dr Ernst's sentence.

On receiving Judge Lutwyche's comments, the colonial secretary, R.G.W. Herbert, submitted the petition to the Executive Council, which rejected it. Towards the end of his sentence Ernst tried again to have his term reduced. In November 1862, Queen Victoria's eldest son, Edward, Prince of Wales, was about to celebrate his twenty-first birthday. On such occasions it was the practice to grant amnesty to selected prisoners. The doctor made a plea to Governor Bowen to exercise the Royal Prerogative to have the remainder of his term remitted. His Excellency took the plea to the Executive Council but the council "failed to perceive any circumstance in Gustav Ernst's case to induce them to advise the special exercise of the Prerogative of Mercy on his behalf". Ernst was obliged to serve another four months to complete his sentence. Encouraged by the earlier petition of the citizens of Musket Flat to have him return to practise among them he decided to remain in the district. A report in the *Brisbane Courier* in 1866 mentions his attending the proprietor of an hotel in Gayndah.

The Unusual Dr Jonathan Labatt

In the early days of medicine in Queensland, doctors mercilessly criticized each other in the press. Statements were made which today would bring censure from the ethics committees, if not libel suits. Usually the arguments went no further than letter-writing, but for one Dr Jonathan Labatt of Warwick, feuding with a fellow doctor and other citizens landed him in jail among the lunatics of Moreton Bay.

Dr Labatt was born in Dublin and graduated from the King's and Queen's College of Physicians in Ireland. He was registered by the New South Wales medical board on 18 May 1852 and went to Warwick shortly afterwards. At first things went well for the Irish graduate. He was appointed medical officer to the Aborigines and also became a magistrate. Socially, he entertained Governor General Fitzroy, and Rev. Glennie states in his diary that "he introduced the bishop to Dr Labatt who conducted him to Maryvale".

But in 1855 Dr Labatt came into collision with Dr Otto Sasche, a German practitioner who had graduated from the University of Berlin. At first Sasche's foreign degree was not recognized by the medical board but that did not stop him putting up his plate. The two medicos were soon at loggerheads. It is difficult to say who was to blame, for both were quick-tempered gentlemen. It was Labatt who probably fired the first public shot in a letter on 5 March in the Sydney paper, *Empire*, under the heading, "Notes from the North" and signed "Correspondent". The article claimed that Sasche was not a duly qualified medical practitioner in Australia and cast doubts on his ability as a doctor. Sasche replied with an advertisement in the *Moreton Bay Courier*, which included a letter of support from thirty-seven citizens, including John Douglas, JP, Rev. T. Kingsford, Rev. Benjm. Glennie and Rev. W. McGinty. Otto Sasche must have gained immediate popularity in Warwick to collect such signatures.

Later in the year, a young man named Lederingham was the victim of an assault and died some days afterwards. He was attended by Dr Sasche. In a letter published in the *Moreton Bay Courier* Dr Labatt said Sasche had bungled the case and had neglected to give treatment "which would have suggested itself to a tyro in a British hospital". Sasche replied a few editions later by saying Labatt had refused to come when called in consultation. Sasche added: "You cannot even pretend to be a surgeon".

Sasche was later recognized by the medical board and went to practise in the Toowoomba-Drayton area. His place in Warwick was taken by Dr Samuel W. Aldred, an English graduate, who was later to become mayor. Aldred in time came to be held in high esteem by the Warwick citizens. But his popularity did not save him from Dr Labatt.

After Dr Sasche's departure, Dr Labatt continued to be in the news. In June 1857, a stack of wheat on his property was burnt down but a store containing corn was saved. He claimed that the fire was deliberately lit and a "train was found leading from the stack to the store". Labatt was also a party in a number of minor court cases and on one occasion he struck Dr Aldred with a whip during an argument. Labatt himself tasted the heavy lash of a whip when he quarrelled with Mr J.W. Buckland, JP.

But in 1861, Dr Labatt's tempestuous nature got him into much deeper trouble. The events which were to have such serious consequences for the doctor were described by Labatt himself:

> On Thursday, the 28th November, 1861, two women of very dissolute character, who resided in the house immediately adjoining mine, and whom I had repeatedly requested Mr Halloran, the magistrate, to take steps to remove, roared out and defied me to go anywhere near their place. I walked over, and one attacked me with a green hide and the other with a small wicket gate. I then walked away, and said, "I shall punish you very severely". They defied me to pass the house again, and when I approached it, they both attacked me again — one with a sapling, an inch and a-half in diameter, and the other with a gate; and on my retreating, I sustained a cut on the head, and in warding off the blows, my arm became as black as my shoe. Shortly after, my extremities became cold, and I was suffering from severe pain in the head, which I attribute to concussion of the brain — more or less, from the blows received. There were several persons outside, who witnessed this assault, among whom was Mr Halloran's son, whom I requested to go for his father; I also sent for Dr Aldred to put some plaster on my head. The chief constable came, and I requested him to go for Mr Halloran, which I presume he did, but Mr Halloran did not attend. On Thursday, that day week, I went to the police office to get a summons against the two women, for this serious assault, and I got the summons the following Wednesday. The Saturday week after I sustained the accident, the 7th. December, 1861, the case was called on, and I asked where was Dr Aldred, who had to give material

> evidence as to the nature of the wounds I had sustained. Mr Halloran said he would go on without him, and I said that I wished to have the case postponed till the Monday next, in order that there should be no mistake. I then went across to Mr Aldred's house, and I was told he would attend in half-an-hour's time. I told Mr Halloran that Dr Aldred would be in court in half-an-hour, but he peremptorily refused to postpone the case, though I had said that I would prefer not entering into the case without the presence of the medical man. On my way to Mr Glennie, on Saturday, 14th, I called at Mr Oxenheim's, the solicitor, and in a most quiet tone of voice asked where my family was; he said that my poor wife had gone to the North, which I afterwards ascertained was not the case. I then said, "I can't believe it, Mr Oxenheim, and it will be my painful duty, if they do not return to their proper home, to caution the public." To which Mr Oxenheim replied, "If you dare to do so I will send you to gaol for six months". I then proceeded to Mr Glennie's and I asked him to go in search of my family, and conjure them to return home, which he kindly promised to do. That day, in the afternoon, I called again on Mr Glennie, but he was out. In the evening, between seven and eight o'clock, having made enquiry for this purpose, I rapped at Mr Oxenheim's door, and asked him where my family was; and he said, "If you don't get agone, I will put you in the lock-up", in the most insulting manner; and that being the second time that day that he had seriously insulted, I was greatly aggrieved. At that time I was under no excitement except the wound. I then broke four or five panes of glass in his French window, and his wife came out; I made a most humble apology, and shook hands with her and gave her to understand I would pay expenses, but her husband had been suborning my family.

Mr Oxenheim was as good as his word. He sent for Chief Constable Watt, who, after observing the broken glass, went in search of Dr Labatt. When Watt found the doctor, he took him in custody as he did not consider him to be of sound mind nor a fit person to be at large. As it was Saturday night, Labatt spent the weekend in the Warwick lockup. On Monday 16 December 1861, he was brought before Arthur Halloran, the police magistrate, St George R. Gore, JP, and another man — J.W. Buckland, JP, — who had previously struck Labatt with a whip in a quarrel. When Chief Constable Watt laid the charge before the bench, he tendered two medical certificates, one from Dr Aldred, whom Labatt had once struck with a whip, and the other from Dr F.N. Lucas, who had recently settled in Warwick after leaving Ipswich. Dr Aldred's certificate stated that he considered Dr Labatt to be of unsound mind, to be dangerous to society and needing restraint. Dr Lucas's certificate supported Dr Aldred

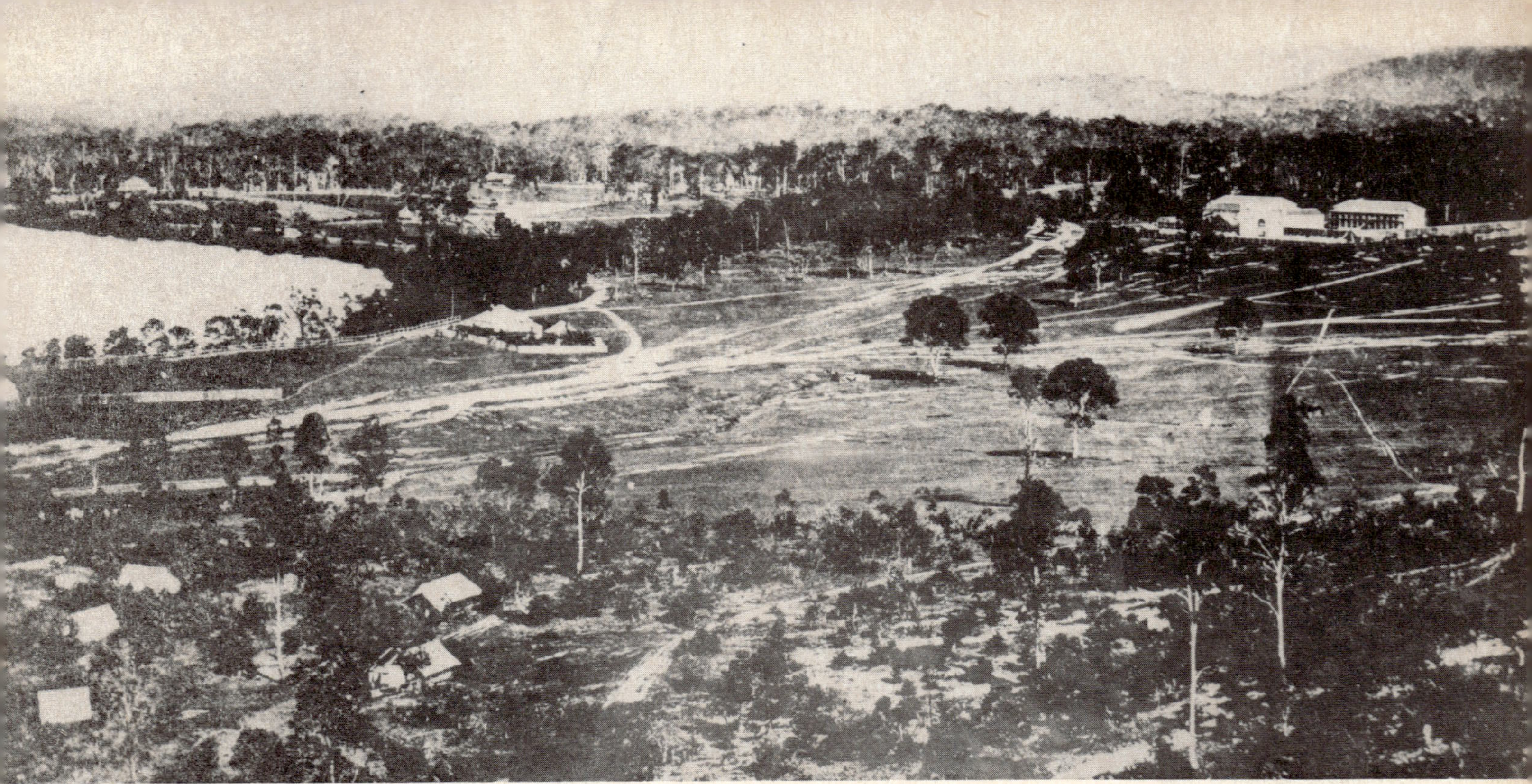

A view of Brisbane in 1862 showing Roma Street and, in the top right, the Brisbane Gaol on Petrie Terrace where the tempestuous Dr Labatt was imprisoned. (Courtesy Oxley Library)

but, curiously, it said that he had not examined Dr Labatt very lately.

The bench committed Labatt and in the warrant commanded the chief constable "to take the said Jonathan Labatt to the said gaol at Brisbane and deliver him in safe custody to the keeper therein". It further commanded the keeper of the said gaol "to receive the said Jonathan Labatt into his custody and keep him in strict custody until the said Jonathan Labatt was discharged by order of the Judge of the Supreme Court of Queensland or until the said Jonathan Labatt was removed to some Lunatic Asylum by order of His Excellency, the Governor of Queensland".

At this time, Queensland had no lunatic asylum, as psychiatric hospitals were called then. While the area was still Moreton Bay and part of New South Wales, lunatics were held in the gaol, or sometimes in the hospital. Meanwhile, a report of the case would be sent by ship to Sydney and a warrant sent back to send the patient to Tarban Creek Lunatic Asylum, the forerunner of Gladesville Psychiatric Hospital. Sir George Ferguson Bowen, the first governor of Queensland, wrote to Governor General William Denison immediately after separation asking for this arrangement to continue, but his request was refused. Until an asylum was opened at Woogaroo west of Brisbane, near present-day Goodna, in January 1865, psychiatric patients were housed in Brisbane Gaol.

And so Dr Labatt was escorted by two constables to Brisbane Gaol, travelling via Toowoomba and Ipswich. The party left Warwick on horseback on 18 December. Bishop Quinn, the first Catholic bishop, accompanied the party for a time, riding alongside Dr Labatt, with the constables some distance behind them. They stopped at Clifton for lunch. A young lady was present during the meal. At first she was apprehensive, but later she was observed sitting alone with Dr Labatt on the verandah. She told Dr Quinn that her early apprehension was not justifiable. The bishop left the party at Etonvale, where Labatt pleaded with the constables to stay the night as he claimed he was exhausted. But the constables were under instructions and took Labatt on to Toowoomba where he spent some time. He was visited by several people who knew him, including his old adversary, Otto Sasche. This article appeared in the *Darling Downs Gazett.*

> The late residents of Warwick, who have settled in Toowoomba, were very much surprised when they were informed that Dr Labatt, who once held in Warwick as a physician and a magistrate a distinguished

> position had arrived at the lockup at Toowoomba escorted by the Police under a charge of being a dangerous lunatic. We are informed that none of the visitors, Dr Sasche, Messers Berkman, McCarthy, Paterson and others could discover any aberration of intellect. Dr Labatt complains that an assault he committed with a stock whip was taken as sufficient cause to detain him as a dangerous lunatic, that he was handcuffed in Warwick, and very badly treated until he arrived here. Measures have been taken to treat him, on his further journey, as a gentleman and with consideration to his advanced age and former standing in society. We are surprised to find Mr Aldred was one of the gentlemen signing the certificate, as cases of insanity belong strictly to the province of a physician and Mr Aldred acted as a physician contrary to the 7th clause of the Queensland Medical Act and made himself liable to a penalty of £20. It would be as well if medical men made themselves acquainted with the Act now in force whereby practitioners acting in other capacity than that for which they are registered are amenable to a penalty.

Leaving Toowoomba, the journey took another two days' riding with Dr Labatt spending an overnight stay in the Ipswich lockup. On Christmas Eve, he was delivered to Samuel Sneyd, the keeper of Brisbane Gaol, still protesting to anyone who would listen that he was not insane.

During this period the gaol population was 101: 78 prisoners and 23 lunatics. Theoretically prisoners and lunatics were separated but this was not so in practice. On arrival everyone was put with the criminals. There was no classification of prisoners, some of whom cared for the lunatics. F.O. Darvall, the visiting justice, said that "in some constitutions, the circumstances would lead to insanity. Confinement in a yard without shelter from the sun, with raving and blaspheming lunatics would drive men of certain constitutions mad".

It was here Dr Labatt spent Christmas, New Year, and the first two weeks of January. Dr Kearsey Cannan, visiting surgeon to the gaol, examined Labatt on admission but took no further action for nearly three weeks. It was Darvall, the visiting justice, who believed that Dr Labatt was not insane, and wrote to the colonial secretary. In his letter of 17 January, he suggested that a medical board of at least two medical gentleman should enquire into the present state of mind of the doctor. Six days later Manning, the principal undersecretary, asked Dr Fullerton, the president of the medical board, to nominate members of a medical commission to examine Dr Labatt. Fullerton, on 27 January, replied to Manning, nominating doctors Cannan, Bell,

Hobbs and himself. This commission did not meet as action had been taken in another quarter. Dr Labatt had written to the governor and it is probably as a result of this that Dr Cannan and Samuel Sneyd submitted certificates to Judge Lutwyche of the Supreme Court, to the effect that Labatt had improved and was fit to be discharged. The judge, under the Lunacy Act Amendment Act of 1845, wrote an order for Labatt's discharge immediately and he was discharged on 23 January 1862, forty days after he was arrested.

For the next three years, Labatt stayed in Brisbane. Darvall, who was registrar-general as well as visiting justice to the gaol, employed him in his office. The only complaint he had about the doctor's behaviour was that he had "a disposition to take part in any conversation that was going on in the room and with persons coming into the room. He would stop work and enter into conversation sometimes disagreeably". He also practised professionally. But, all the time, he attempted to obtain redress for what he considered was the dreadful wrong done to him. He brought an action in law against the magistrates who had committed him. Halloran, the police magistrate, instructed the chief constable not to serve the writ as he claimed it was disrespectful for the officer to serve writs against magistrates under whom he served and that it was the duty of the bailiff at Toowoomba to perform this task. When the bailiff did serve the writ and the matter was brought to a hearing, the case was thrown out on a technicality. The attorney's name and address were not on the writ. Dr Labatt had to pay £20 costs of court and his solicitor's fees.

The doctor wrote numerous letters to Mr R.G.W. Herbert, the colonial secretary, and succeeded in obtaining an interview with him, but all to no avail. Interestingly, he applied for the position of superintendent of the asylum that the government was now building at Woogaroo. He was unsuccessful, the position going to Dr Cannan, the man who had first examined him at the gaol. Finally he petitioned parliament and succeeded in having a select committee, consisting of Dr Challinor, chairman, and Lilley, Bell, Douglas and Kennedy, to enquire into his case. It was not until September 1864 that its report was tabled in the house.

1. The labours of your committee have been chiefly directed to the history of the case, from Dr Labatt's removal from Warwick to his discharge from the asylum by order of Mr Justice Lutwyche, as there was no evidence available to your committee respecting occurrences prior to his removal, except that of two of the committing Magistrates.

2. The whole of the witnesses examined with regard to the period referred to above, admit that Dr Labatt suffered more or less during that interval from mental excitement, but they were also unanimous in their opinion that that mental excitement might be fairly attributed to other causes than of insanity. The evidence of Dr Fullerton, and his letter to Dr Labatt, dated October 28th, 1863, and which will be found in the Appendix, are very explicit as to one of the alleged causes of that excitement.
3. Your committee is of the opinion that, in all cases of mental derangement brought under the notice of benched Magistrates, it would be well to adopt the course pursued in New South Wales, — namely, to bind the offending party to keep the peace and failing to find sureties, to deal with him as in ordinary cases of like default.
4. Your committee cannot conclude its report without expressing its deep regret any circumstances should have arisen necessitating the enquiry referred to them by your Honourable House.

During the evidence, Darvall, the visiting justice, said he considered Labatt to be eccentric; Sneyd, the keeper of the gaol, and Gillan, the principal turnkey, both thought his excitement was due to delirium tremens; Bishop Quinn said that "Labatt was in as equable a state of mind as anyone, under the circumstances, could be expected to be". Dr Fullerton's letter, referred to in the report, contained these words:

> I recollect that my first interview with you was when you called at my house in February, 1862, and neither on that occasion, nor during our acquaintance since, did I discover any symptom of lunacy, nor have I heard any reason why you should have been confined as a lunatic.
>
> From the report I received from yourself, or aught gleaned from other sources, I am obliged to look upon your confinement in prison as an exercise of arbitrary power too gross to be sanctioned in any civilized community.

Despite the report there is no evidence that Dr Labatt received any direct compensation. However, in 1865 he was appointed superintendent of the Benevolent Asylum at Dunwich. This appointment may be taken as a gesture by the government to make amends for the treatment he had received. But he was not long out of trouble. Part of his duty was to visit St Helena Island, where the quarantine station was situated, and off which the prison hulk, *Proserpine*, was moored. On 16 February 1866, the sick attendant found Dr Labatt on his bed in his tent, too drunk to attend to the sick. Five days later, his servant reported that he was missing. Staff from the prison hulk, and the prisoners, searched the island. He was found, dressed only in his shirt, and badly bitten by mosquitoes. He said he had had an appointment with a friend but some young fellow had stolen his clothes. John McDonald, the officer in charge of the police on the hulk, reported the incident to R.R. McKenzie, who was now the colonial secretary, and Dr Labatt was told his services were no longer required. Dr Labatt wrote to the colonial secretary, beginning with these words: "I understand I have incurred your displeasure. If such is the case I greatly regret it but confidently trust you will suspend your opinion, in justice to me, until my return to Brisbane, where I am sure I shall have no difficulty in relieving your mind from any unfavourable impression it may entertain respecting me." His pleading was to no avail.

Dr Labatt returned to Warwick, where he died in 1869. Douglas Gordon, commenting on his obituary, said that it was "correct and proper, but short and unenthusiastic".

Birth of a Hospital

> To relieve the poor, the distressed and the aged and thereby to discountenance as much as possible, mendacity and vagrancy and to encourage industrious habits among the indigent as well as to afford them religious instruction and consolation in distress.

Thus were expressed the objectives of the Moreton Bay Benevolent Society formed at a general meeting of inhabitants of the district held at the Court House, Brisbane on 14 October 1844. The meeting elected as officers of the society, Captain Wickham, the police magistrate, president; David Ballow, assistant colonial surgeon, treasurer; and Louis Layard, secretary. Among the rules adopted by the newly-formed society was a stipulation that relief should generally not be afforded in money, but in needed articles. Only in exceptional cases would money be given as relief. One interesting rule gave free membership to ministers who preached a collection sermon for the society once every six months, and to those Brisbane medical gentlemen who gave their services gratuitously. Others who desired membership were obliged to subscribe £1 per annum. For £30 they were rewarded with the society's life membership.

While the wording of the objectives and rules, and even the purport of the rules themselves, may appear quaint to present-day readers, the society was sincere in its efforts to relieve distress in a community which provided no other social services. It provided outdoor relief — helping destitute families — and paid for hospitalization. When the latter was achieved the society — perhaps for publicity, or perhaps for pride in its work — published the details in the *Moreton Bay Courier*. In those days people were apparently less easily offended, for in one report concerning eighteen people that it had helped by paying the hospital bill were the following details.

> No. 11 John Groves, syphilis; admitted 25th Jan, discharged 21st March.
>
> No. 12 John Williams, suppression urinae; admitted 7th Feb, discharged 21st March.
>
> No. 15 George Horne, gonorrhea; admitted 5th March, discharged 27th March.

The hospital in which the society arranged treatment for these men was the convict hospital — Her Majesty's General Hospital, Moreton Bay. Although the penal settlement had closed and free settlement begun, the government was obliged to provide medical treatment for the military detachment, prisoners and officials who remained. Others who sought admission were the poor free settlers who had no home in which to be nursed. David Ballow, the surgeon, saw the need for medical services to be provided for others besides those who had an official claim, and he wrote to his superiors in Sydney for advice. Early in 1842, the year the district was thrown open to free settlement, he advised the director general of hospital services that he considered that Moreton Bay had become like any other part of the colony and asked whether private individuals and assigned prisoners could be admitted. He was told that the masters of assigned prisoners were to be charged one shilling a day for hospitalization, but no paupers were to be admitted without the previous order of the government, except in cases of accident or emergency. The surgeon in charge would be considered personally responsible for any expense incurred in contravention of these orders. Free settlers were charged three shillings a day. But, before admission, they needed two responsible and substantial householders to guarantee before a police magistrate or justice of the peace that they would pay the bill. Bonds, such as the one following, appear in the records.

> We hereby bind ourselves to pay the expenses of the medical treatment of James Smith in Her Majesty's Hospital at Brisbane Town, Moreton Bay and in the event of his death to defray the expenses of his interment.

The illnesses for which treatment was sought were of a medical but not surgical nature. Besides the venereal diseases which figured in the report of the Moreton Bay Benevolent Society, Dr Ballow diagnosed rheumatism and intermittent fever in many who asked for his aid. Many medical writers have suggested that the intermittent fever was malaria. This may be so, but often it was probably what was called in later years the "flu". It was to be several years before the abdomen was opened for surgical conditions and the scalpel was used mostly for amputations, the letting of blood, and the draining of pus. When the *Sovereign* was wrecked in 1847 in Moreton Bay the survivors who had been washed ashore after the terrible ordeal were treated at the hospital. In the same year two sawyers, Boller and Smith, were speared by Aborigines while cutting timber at North Pine. Knight, in his book *In the Early Days*, said that the two were at first refused admission because they did not have guarantors. A good Samaritan later came along and promised all dues. He met these claims and also defrayed the funeral expenses for Boller, who died from his wounds.

Although Dr Ballow had been given permission to admit free settlers, he was also advised of the government's desire to close the hospital now that the penal settlement had ceased to function. He sought Wickham's help and the two managed to keep the hospital open for another six years. In support of his pleas, Ballow pointed out to Sydney that the hospital was essential for the treatment of the intermittent fever among prisoners at Limestone (Ipswich) and for the many accident cases which occurred. Finally, its doom was sealed early in 1848 when Ballow received an order for its closure that he could not refuse. Despite the knowledge that such an event was always imminent the inhabitants of Brisbane were outraged. The *Moreton Bay Courier* took the government to task in these words:

> Our humane and tender-hearted Government sent by the last steamer a peremptory order for the discharge of the patients lying in the General Hospital on the 31st ultimo. They were accordingly turned out of the building to seek refuge in the hour of their distress wherever they could on Monday last. Some of the poor creatures could scarcely crawl, and it was really pitiable to witness their sufferings on the occasion. Had it not been for the kindness and humanity of some of the inhabitants several might have perished in the streets. Considering that the Government does not require the use of the building for present purposes, it would have been more consonant with the dictates of humanity to have allowed the poor people to remain until they were convalescent; and to have given directions that no more patients should be admitted after a certain date; provision could then have been made for the future. The conduct of Government in this affair has been neither humane nor decorous; a private individual would be ashamed of it. But they have ordered every gallipot and phial with their contents to be packed up in readiness for transmission to Sydney.

The closure brought quick and sensible action from Wickham. He wrote to the colonial secretary, pointing out the great inconvenience to the settlement that had occurred and asked that a portion of the hospital be retained for the treatment of patients willing to pay and those whose expenses were defrayed by the Benevolent Society. He asked for a government subsidy for a hospital committee, as had been given to other centres. The colonial secretary met Wickham's request. In fact, he expressed willingness to hand over the whole of the building and its facilities. The Moreton Bay settlement was fortunate. It would have a hospital already built, albeit a little in need of repair. Other settlements had to erect their own hospital. The *Moreton Bay Courier*, which had slated the government for closing the hospital, now praised its generous action in handing over the whole of the building with its furniture and instruments and the promise of a £200 per annum subsidy, providing a similar sum could be raised by a committee.

The following months were busy ones. The necessary committee was formed to take advantage of the government's offer. At its request, the *Moreton Bay Courier* published an article addressed to shepherds, hutkeepers and others engaged in pastoral pursuits in the Moreton Bay and Darling Downs districts, soliciting subscriptions. The paper submitted that the contributions should be general — not confined to one particular class — so townspeople as well as bushmen could combine to promote the project. It quoted a celebrated author who had said that "the race of mankind would perish did they cease to aid each other. From the time the mother binds the child's head till the moment that some kind assistant wipes the death damp from the brow of the dying, we cannot exist without mutual help. All therefore, that need aid, have a right to ask for it from their fellow mortals; no man who holds the power of granting can refuse it without guilt". The paper then exhorted the shepherds, hutkeepers and others engaged in the pastoral industry to contibute ten shillings towards the hospital. Most in the settlement agreed that two committees whose objectives were much the same were too much for the community and so the Benevolent Society agreed to disband and hand over its funds of £75.5s.8d to the hospital committee. A further step was necessary. Legislation required that the property be vested in trustees. A meeting of the steering committee elected the following: Doctors David Ballow and Stephen Simpson, and Messrs J. Richardson, W. Pickering and G.S. Le Breton.

On 3 October 1848, David Ballow, on behalf of the trustees, and Lieutenant Colonel J.A. Gordon, on behalf of the government, signed an historic document by which the hospital buildings and contents were delivered to the Moreton Bay Hospital Committee. Although the hospital started to take patients on 6 November 1848 when Phillip Corbett, an eighty-year-old pauper suffering from an ulcer, was admitted, it was put on an official basis on 12 January 1849 when the first annual meeting was held. The meeting elected Captain Wickham as president, with William Duncan becoming the first treasurer, and William Wilkes the secretary. The committee appointed David Ballow, who had resigned from the colonial medical service, as house surgeon, and Kearsey Cannan as visiting surgeon. The meeting also adopted twenty-three rules to guide the committee in the administration of the hospital. The first rule contained the hospital objectives, which read not unlike those of the Benevolent Society: "To relieve the poor, the distressed and the aged and to afford them religious instruction and consolation". There was no mention of nursing the sick. The committee strived to achieve its objectives but they were objectives that placed on it a heavy burden for many years to come. An allied rule empowered the committee to defray the cost of the passage of destitute persons to Sydney. Any person who subscribed £1 per annum became a member and life membership was awarded to those who donated £10 in one payment. Members enjoyed the privilege of recommending one patient for admission or six to the dispensary. Before admission, a charge of three shillings a day had to be guaranteed by a bond entered into by one or more responsible persons, or the lodgment of the expected cost with the treasurer. Paupers were admitted on the recommendation of a member provided the committee was completely satisfied that the person was totally unable to defray expenses. If the pauper had any property he or she was obliged to deliver it to the committee to pay expenses. In a letter advising Ballow of his appointment as house surgeon, the secretary stated that the smallness of his salary of £25 per annum and house was occasioned solely by funds available. He was allowed two full diets for his servants. The secretary's commiseration did not satisfy Kearsey Cannan, who declined the position when he was advised that his salary as visiting surgeon would be £30 per annum. When the committee found another £20 per annum, he accepted.

The greatest problem the committee had to face was that which plagues every hospital management — finance, or rather the lack of it. The committee needed funds for the everyday care of the sick and the destitute; for the repairs to the hospital, and later for additions. Care of the destitute included outdoor relief as well as hospitalization. The minutes of the committee meetings show how seriously it took its objective of caring for the destitute. At its meeting on 28 March 1850, the committee noted that Mary

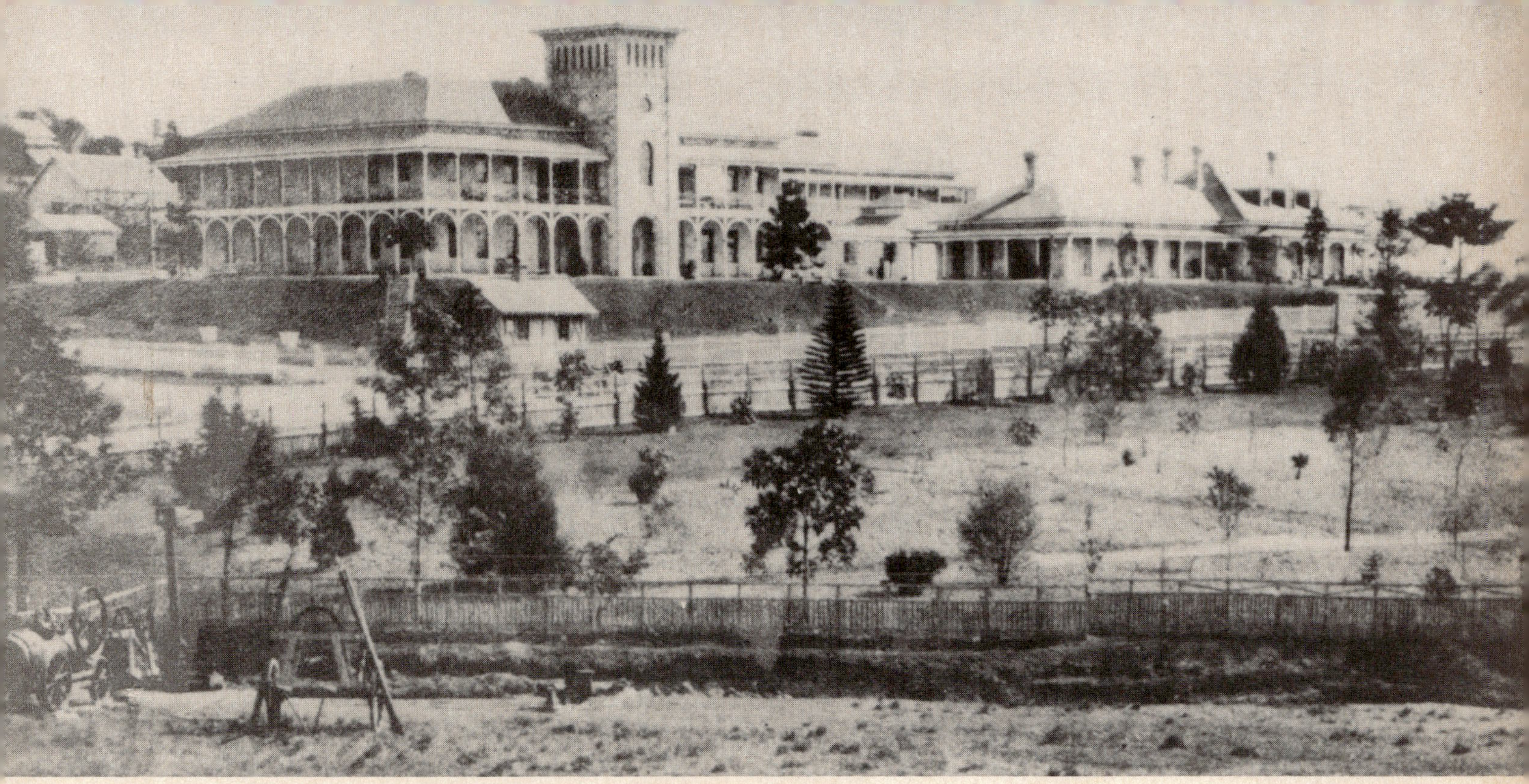

The "new" Brisbane Hospital (c1876) on Bowen Bridge Road was built by John Petrie and was first occupied in 1867. It is now the site of the Royal Brisbane Hospital. (Courtesy Oxley Library)

Fallon, a pauper, who with two children had been admitted to hospital, should be allowed to stay a few days longer, to see if she improved enough to be discharged. Two weeks later, it was agreed that she should stay another seven days and then be allowed a fortnight's rations as well as her rent being paid by the committee for a month after she left hospital. In one case, the committee defrayed the expenses of a patient who was sent to Sydney to attend an eye specialist, Dr Berncastle.

In 1844, Ballow had advised his superior in Sydney that the roof needed shingling, wards were in need of repair, plaster was falling from the ceiling, and panes of glass were deficient. These had not been attended to when the civilian committee assumed charge. The chronically ill and the destitute were long-stay cases and greatly overtaxed the accommodation. The position became so desperate that temporary accommodation was provided elsewhere for the benevolent cases before further wards were added.

The committee had sources other than subscriptions, some of them interesting. Under legislation called Lord Lansdowne's Act, benevolent societies could claim money paid in fines for drunkenness, common assault and malicious injury to property. The Moreton Bay Benevolent Society's right to claim such fines was transferred to the hospital committee and the benches were notified accordingly. The efforts of the treasurer to collect the fines were worthwhile as the amounts involved were not inconsiderable. In 1851, he received £63 from this source when the cost of running the hospital for the year was approximately £400. The Brisbane bench forwarded the moneys promptly but some of the country clerks of the courts were very tardy in fulfilling this duty. The correspondence indicates that money was sometimes used for other official purposes and sometimes it appears that the clerks may have pocketed it themselves. William Duncan once wrote to the clerk at Warwick in a private capacity to tell the clerk that his cheque had been dishonoured. When this matter was at last raised officially, Duncan was most indignant that his well-meant, gratuitous hint had not only been ignored but that he was accused by the country official of being in error. From time to time, churches held special services at which the collections were donated to the hospital. The following extract is taken from a letter written in 1851 to seven ministers in Brisbane asking them to preach on a suitable day. Its wording indicates that the hopes the *Moreton Bay Courier* expressed in 1848 that donations would be forthcoming from shepherds, hutkeepers and others engaged in the pastoral pursuits were fruitless.

> Since the establishment of this institution it has constantly been found that the labouring men throughout these districts have, whilst in health evinced the utmost indifference to the prosperity of the hospital and have utterly failed to give the smallest assistance to the funds from the large wages they have hitherto enjoyed and the savings from which they appear to have, felt far greater pleasure in spending in drunkenness and dissipation as injurious to their morals as destructive to their health but when the consequences of such conduct have manifested themselves in poverty and disease and those thoughtless and mistaken men have no refuge but this institution from starvation and death; and have been but too happy to avail themselves of the funds collected with extreme difficulty from others more benevolent and less culpable.

The letter then went on to say that a sermon that would loosen the pursestrings of such men would be appropriate.. Three parsons responded to the request, but no account of the result has been found.

The good ladies of Brisbane often rallied to the cause of the hospital. They excelled themselves in 1858 when a bazaar and a ball realized £658, no mean sum for the time. Although the government's expressed philosophy was that the community should manage the hospital, it was, in fact, quite generous when special need arose. The government also paid for repairs when the committee could not. The money raised by the ladies' bazaar and ball was used to match £800 promised by the government for additional accommodation for the benevolent patients. The difficulty in raising funds influenced the attitude of the Brisbane committee in 1856 when it heard that the citizens of Ipswich were endeavouring to establish a hospital in that town. Realizing that such a move would deprive it of subscribers and the fines from the Ipswich bench, a special meeting was called. The committee asked the colonial secretary in Sydney if a copy of the memorial from Ipswich could be sent before any action was taken by the government. Not surprisingly, the colonial secretary declined the request. After separation in 1859, the Queensland government continued to subsidize the funds raised by the committee. In 1865, it provided £2,500 — £1,000 for the hospital and £1,500 for the upkeep of benevolent patients.

Serious attempts were also made to provide religious instruction for the patients. When the number of visiting surgeons was increased, the committee allotted each patient a surgeon and a minister of religion on admission. The ministers attended regularly and on occasions the ladies came also to give spiritual

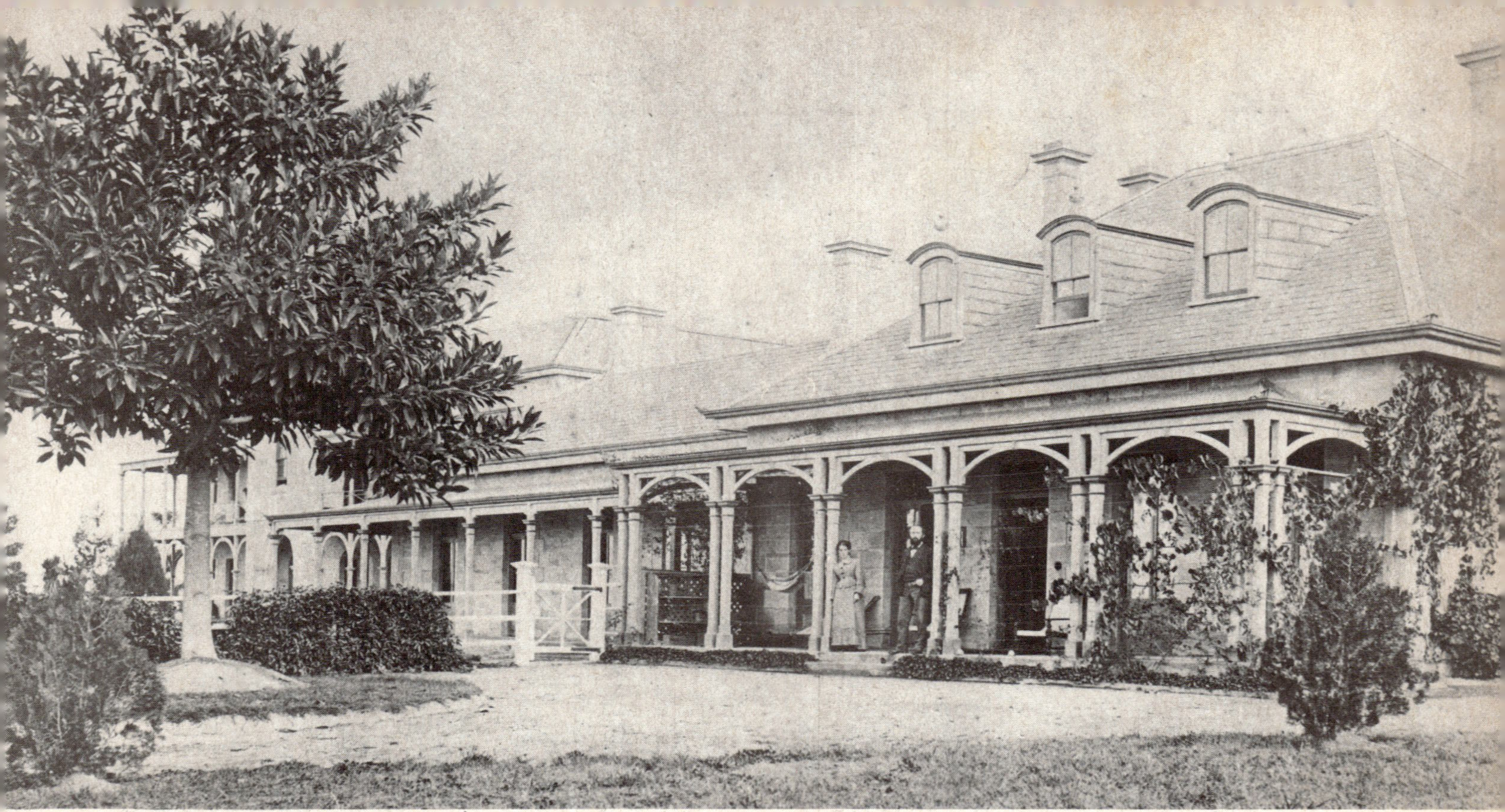

The Brisbane Hospital superintendent lived in this house next to the hospital. The superintendent from 1876 to 1882, Dr John Thomson, is pictured on the verandah with his wife. (Courtesy Oxley Library)

help. However, when one enthusiastic parson held divine service in a ward and exposed members of other flocks as well as his own to his sermon, he was severely reprimanded by the committee.

When David Ballow, the first house surgeon, died from typhus fever at Dunwich in 1850, Frederick Barton, who had come to help in the epidemic, was appointed in his stead at the hospital. After two years in the post, Barton left the hospital to conduct a pharmacy in Queen Street and there advertised that he would perform bleeding, cupping and the drawing of teeth. Hugh Bell carried on the duties of house surgeon, and then Barton gave up the pharmacy and returned to the hospital, staying until 1863. Then John Lansdowne was appointed to take charge of the institution. When a select committee was appointed in 1866 to enquire into hospitals in the colony, Lansdowne drew attention to the poor standard of nursing at the hospital. Apart from the lack of training, the nurses were expected to sleep in the wards. Lansdowne stated that this prevented the type of women he would like to see appointed from applying for the positions.

In time, the objective of helping the destitute became harder to meet. Despite the additional accommodation, overcrowding in the benevolent wing increased and the financial burden was too much for the committee. The government was approached with a view to separating the hospital and benevolent patients. Robert Herbert, the colonial secretary, attended the annual meeting in 1864 and the committee was delighted to hear him announce that both institutions should be moved to the suburbs and that the government and the committee would jointly choose a new site for the hospital. Their delight turned to concern when it was rumoured the government had already chosen a site. This was indeed true. Executive records show that not only had a site been chosen without consulting the hospital committee, but it had been chose on 31 December 1863, two weeks before Herbert announced that the selection of a site would be a joint effort. The record also shows that Charles Tiffin, the colonial architect, had been instructed to draw plans for a new hospital on 15 acres at Bowen Bridge in the vicinity of the local municipal council's acclimatization gardens. The committee wrote to the colonial secretary, stating that if this were indeed the site, there were strong objections, particularly in regard to the distance from the town. An alternative site was suggested near the fever hospital, which incidentally the government had built, at Green Hills, near Countess Street and Roma Street. This was the beginning of several months' wrangling during which another site at York's

Hollow, where Gilchrist Avenue now runs, was considered and rejected. Finally, the government ended the dispute with the following letter.

> These matters have had frequent consideration by the Government and as the result of their deliberation I am to state that it is proposed to establish the principal hospital on the site chosen near Bowen Bridge. The Government will be happy to relieve the committee from all connection with it should they so desire or will be willing to appoint a visiting committee not responsible for the details of management.

The committee admitted defeat in a letter that suggested that its obligations were the reason for doing so.

> The committee do not desire neither do they consider that they have any power to relieve themselves of the responsibility which devolves on them by virtue of their election by the governors of the Hospital.

Tiffin, the architect, had planned a four hundred-bed hospital and a contract was let for a one hundred-bed section. The first contractor, William Robertson, failed to meet conditions and John Petrie, whose skill can still be seen in many buildings in Brisbane, took over. During excavations, Petrie's men found the fossilized remains of a prehistoric animal. When it was exhibited later, a newspaper report read: "Alexander McPherson exhibited a part of an immense fossil found whilst blasting out the foundations of the Brisbane Hospital. Mr McPherson considers it the fossil of a huge reptile, and estimates its length at thirty-five feet and its diameter could be traced in the rock some six or seven feet. A great portion of this interesting specimen was buried in a heap of rubbish by the workmen, who were ignorant of its value; but Mr McPherson managed to secure about three tons weight. He has informed us that a bank of fossils runs right through Bowen Park."

Petrie finished the contract ahead of time at the end of 1866. The main structure was a two-storeyed, four-ward, stone complex with a central tower. The tower was not an ornament, for it held an overhead tank to which water was pumped from a 36,000 gallon underground tank. From the overhead tank there was a sufficient head of water to flush "proper patent waterclosets" in each ward. There was as yet no connection to the water supply from the Enoggera Reservoir which had begun to flow to the town in July 1866. Although the size of the wards did not allow the standard amount of air space for each patient, Tiffin held that the height of fourteen feet and the ventilation from the spacious verandahs compensated for this deficiency. Each of the large wards held twenty patients, and smaller wards brought the total accommodation to the one hundred beds in the contract. A fever ward also had been built at the rear of the main block. The new hospital included separate accommodation for nurses — a feature that was expected to attract a "better class" of woman. Further features were a mortuary and an operating room with a skylight.

The move to the new hospital was made on 8 January 1867 and was described in the *Brisbane Courier*:

> Yesterday the patients in the old hospital were removed to the new building, on the Bowen Bridge Road, which was handed over to the Government by Mr Petrie, before Christmas, and a considerable time before the contract time had expired. Mr Ebenston accepted the contract for the removal of the patients and the old hospital furniture, which will for the present be used in the new building. The patients, to the number of eighty, were safely conveyed in cabs and carriages, under the superintendence of Dr Lansdowne. They did not seem to be at all the worse for their journey; and they expressed great satisfaction at the additional accommodation provided for them. We have been requested to state that out-door patients will in future have to attend at the new hospital at 10 o'clock every morning.

Gulf Fever

Probably the best known of the expeditions made by HMS *Beagle* was the five year survey voyage in 1831–36 along the South American coast in which Charles Darwin travelled as naturalist. John Clements Wickham, second-in-command of the *Beagle* during the South American voyage with Darwin, later commanded the vessel while charting the northwestern coast of Australia from 1837 to 1841. Wickham retired from the navy and became, firstly, police magistrate at Moreton Bay when the district was thrown open to free settlement in 1842, and, later, government resident. John Lort Stokes, Wickham's lieutenant, succeeded to the command of the *Beagle* when his superior left the brig. Between June and August 1841, Stokes surveyed part of the Gulf of Carpentaria. Whenever possible, Stokes made exploration excursions inland, sometimes reporting enthusiastically on the area he traversed. He travelled up the Albert River for fifty miles by boat and then walked over some of the surrounding country. The following extracts are taken from Stokes's *Discoveries in Australia*, published in London in 1846.

> A vast boundless plain lay before us, here and there dotted over with woodland isles . . . The soil was still a light-coloured mould to great depth and according to one so well qualified to judge as Sir W. Hooker, who kindly examined some that I brought to England, is of a rich quality, confirming the opinion entertained of it, which suggested for this part of the continent, the name of "The Plains of Promise" . . .
>
> We were now once more stepping over a "terra incognita"; and though no alpine features greeted our eyes as they wandered eagerly over the last level, all was clothed in the charm of novelty. The feelings of delight which are naturally aroused in those whose feet for the first time press a new and rich country and which I have so often before endeavoured in vain to express, burst forth on this occasion with renewed intensity . . . Proceeding a little farther, we observed a small lake bearing north half a mile. Attracting by the vernal tints on its border we went to taste the water . . .
>
> All I could do was to give one long lingering look to the southward before I returned. In that direction, however, no curling smoke denoted the presence of the savage; all was lonely and still; and yet even in these deserted plains, equally wanting in the redundance of

> animal, as in the luxuriance of vegetable life, I could discover the rudiments of a future prosperity and ample justification of the name I had bestowed on them. I gazed around, despite my personal disappointment, with feelings of hopeful gratitude to Him who had spread out so fair a dwelling place for creatures; and could not refrain from breathing a prayer that ere long the now level horizon would be broken by a succession of tapering spires rising from the many christian hamlets that must ultimately stud the country, and pointing through the calm depths of the intensely blue and gloriously bright skies of Tropical Australia, to a still calmer and brighter and more glorious region beyond, to which all our sublimest aspirations tend and when our holiest desires may be satisfied.

Four years later Ludwig Leichhardt was in the same area about the same time of the year. The German-born explorer had left Jimbour station on the Darling Downs in October 1844 for Port Essington, near the present site of Darwin. In his diary on 6 August 1845, Leichhardt recorded the windings of a river which he believed was the Albert of Captain Stokes, and the Malt Suyker of the Dutch navigators. Whilst the German explorer did not wax as eloquent as Stokes in his description of the surrounding country, his report would certainly not have discouraged would-be settlers. He reported that the "grass was excellent" and the fresh grass of recent burnings extended all over the plains. He said that the "bright verdure made us believe that we were approaching a fresh water swamp". Whilst he noted that some creeks were dry, there appeared to be sufficient water, and game was plentiful.

The next explorer in the region was A.C. Gregory, who had been chosen to lead an expedition to northern Australia sponsored by the British government. He passed through the Gulf country in August and September 1856, and gave a report very different from the glowing account of Stokes. Gregory said the country around the Gulf did not offer any great inducement to the settler, and he believed the area would be like the Australian inland and be subject to drought. He also claimed that Leichhardt was mistaken, that what he thought was the Albert was an unnamed stream which Gregory then named the Leichhardt. His journal shows that he left the Albert River on 3 September and traversed a level open country thinly clothed with indifferent grass. The land east of the Leichhardt was nearly destitute of grass. However, he did report an improvement in the country as he neared the Flinders. Gregory has been described as modest and unromantic and not one to dramatize what was probably one of the most successful expeditions in the history of Australian exploration. For this reason it seems that the land-hungry pastoralists ignored his warnings.

The next on the scene was William Landsborough. He had been chosen to lead one of the many search parties for Burke and Wills, who had failed to return from the expedition from Melbourne to the Gulf of Carpentaria. Landsborough's pen picture of the country that he traversed in his search from the Gulf southwards resembled that painted by Stokes. In his journal published in 1862, he said the Albert River was surrounded by fine dry plains that were covered with good grasses and they were well suited for sheep runs. He found that horses he had left running near Frost's Ponds were doing well as the herbage in the neighbourhood was of the most fattening kind.

The land seekers in the young colony of Queensland accepted the favourable reports of the Gulf country, and from the end of 1864 mobs of cattle and sheep were driven to the "Plains of Promise" and stations set up. The journal of the Royal Geographical Society referred to the development in the district:

> Sir George Bowen, the active and enlightened Governor of Queensland, has transmitted to us, through the Colonial Office, an account of the establishment of a township near the shores of the Gulf of Carpentaria, being the first settlement made in this fertile and promising region. It is situated at the head of the navigation of the Albert River, and has been named Burketown, in honour of the gallant but unfortunate explorer who lost his life in recrossing the continent of Australia in 1861. The district of Burketown is being rapidly occupied by pastoral settlers who drive their stock overland from the older districts of the colony, but who will receive their supplies chiefly by ships sent around Cape York to the new port of Burketown.

The part played by the government was the appointment of officials to maintain law and order at Burketown. It selected William Landsborough as police magistrate, George Phillips as government surveyor, and young Wentworth Darcy Uhr as officer in charge of the native police. Landsborough set out to travel to his new post on horseback during the summer months of 1865–66. For two years good progress had been made in the area before Landsborough arrived. Lambings were good and wool was being shipped south. Then the gloss began to fade. There were several reasons for this. The first cause for the worsening change was an epidemic of serious fever which killed many in the new district. Then the settlers realized that their remoteness was bringing severe hardships. Essential supplies were at an almost prohibitive price and likewise the cost of sending out the wool was an enormous drain on their finances. Gregory's prediction that the district might be subject to bad seasons came true and the financial crisis that affected the whole colony in 1866–67 caused a lack of the funds so necessary to develop new areas.

One of the earliest reports of the fever appeared in the *Port Denison Times*, Bowen, which published a letter from a correspondent in Burketown in its issue of 16 June 1866. Part of the letter read:

> As is the case in all new settlements, I am sorry to record that fever has been prevalent here, and, in fact, in all new country lately taken up for some time; and deaths from that cause here on different stations now amount to thirty-two.
>
> The disease being so simple, viz., gastric fever which can be readily cured in 24 hours, if taken in time, but if allowed to run on without being checked turns to typhoid, or continued fever, or better known to up-country people as low fever, leads me to suppose that a scarcity of medicine or ignorance of the treatment of the disease on the various stations are the leading causes of so great mortality; especially when you consider the insidious cause of low fever which is rarely understood by persons attacked and seldom attended to at first, most people being averse to taking medicines until really ill.
>
> It is but fair to Burketown to state that the majority of the fatal cases were men who came there sick from the different stations in the hope of obtaining some relief, and who, travelling in a state of fever in a hot climate rendered their cases almost incurable from the lamentable state of weakness to which they were reduced before arriving within reach of medical treatment.
>
> For the information of your country readers I may state that the treatment of the disease on its first appearance is a strong emetic and purgative medicine to follow.

Landsborough, accompanied by Phillips and Uhr, arrived at Burketown in the midst of the epidemic. He described the conditions he found in a letter to Governor Bowen. He found almost everyone in the township sick, and a large number of the original inhabitants had already succumbed to the disease. Phillips, the surveyor, and all of his staff were stricken with the malady and one member had already died. Landsborough reported that no station with which he had any acquaintance had escaped. He stated that he had avoided an attack by moving daily from place to place, but his companions had not been so fortunate. At first, he set up headquarters fourteen miles up the Albert River from the township and gave orders for the police force to remove to the

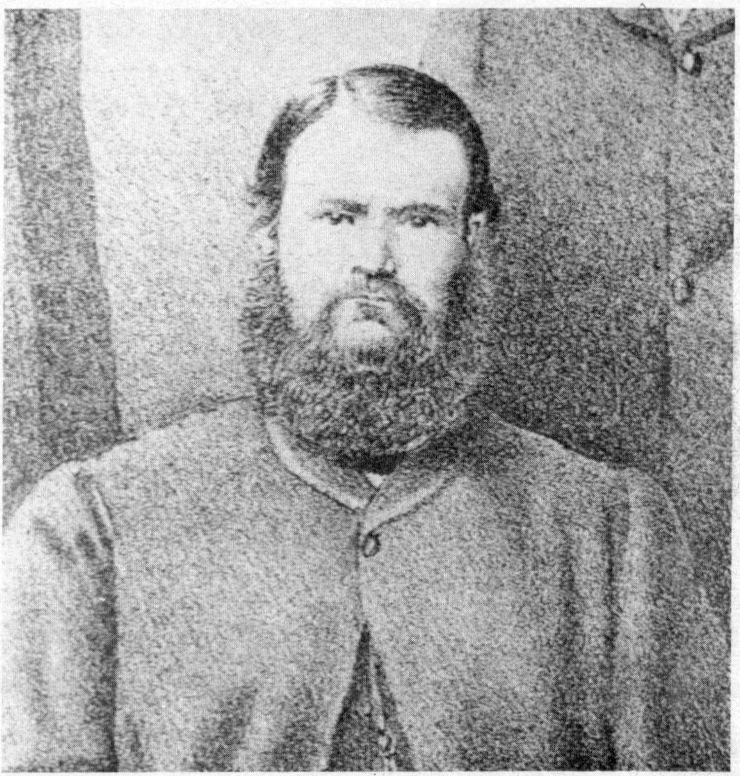

William Landsborough (around 1862), police magistrate in Burketown, Gulf of Carpentaria. (Courtesy Oxley Library)

spot also. Then he decided to move to Sweers Island, about twenty-five miles out to sea from the mouth of the Albert River. All who were able to leave the township were most willing to go with Landsborough to the island. After recounting these experiences, Landsborough expressed the hope that Governor Bowen would visit the area when he made his next northern tour.

The correspondent to the *Port Denison Times*, who had diagnosed and prescribed for the fever, criticized Landsborough's transfer to Sweers Island, saying that many intending settlers had been awaiting the arrival of the new police magistrate with the expectation of receiving some information, however meagre, that might guide them in commencing improvements. Many had travelled long distances to lodge applications with him and then had had to return disappointed. Disputes arising from people erecting shanties on neighbouring runs, being ignorant of the boundaries set aside by the government, remained unsolved.

Duncan McIntyre, the leader of an expedition sponsored by a Melbourne ladies committee to search for Leichhardt, also arrived in the area during the fever epidemic. He gave his version of the tragedy in a letter to his uncle. It was the last letter the explorer wrote, for he too became a victim of the disease. It read:

> We reached the settled districts, Kennedy and McDonald being the furthest out on the Leichhardt. We still kept to the river until we passed the next station, forty miles lower down. We then left it and struck out north-west, and in fifty miles arrived at T.B. McDonald's on the Gregory. Here we were informed of the unhealthiness of the climate — a man having died a few days before our arrival. His grave was quite close to a bit of a shed they called a hut. There being only one on the station, he could not carry his unfortunate companion to any distance. We kept on down the river and in due time arrived at what is called the township or port. The population was about sixty, forty-five or fifty being bad with the fever. In fact, people were sick everywhere. I could not count ten able to do anything in the shape of work. I camped at a lagoon about a mile from the town thinking that I was away from all the sickness. There were a few tents near us. Next morning one of the men in the tents was dead and on going up to the township to get stores I was told that two men had died that morning. I got my stores and started up here, sixteen miles higher up. While putting them in order for packing on the horses, one of the blackboys got the fever and this morning McLeod has got it. The blackboy, I think will get over it, but McLeod thinks it is all over with him. I am well, only waiting for the men to recover. I hope that in a few days they will get better. It does not last long: in one week one is either in his grave or well again. Before I came here there were about eighty in town, sixty-six of whom were bad with the fever. I am told that twenty-five is all that have died in the town, and they are making coffins for two men who are past recovery. I hope that I will get away all right. People are leaving by sea and land as fast as they can. There are two stores — flour, tea and sugar in abundance, but of very bad quality — the flour we can hardly eat it is quite sour — and two public-houses. The present site of the town is on a plain only a few feet above the level of the sea. Perhaps, there is something unusual in the atmosphere this season, but the natives in the country appear to be all right.

About two weeks after McIntyre wrote the letter, Sloman, the second-in-command of the expedition, also wrote to the ladies committee to inform them that "our leader is no more". During the last two days of his life the fever had made McIntyre speechless and "without the slightest of motion". Occasionally he suffered severe pain, while at other times he was at comparative ease. He was buried on 6 June 1866, with Sloman reading the funeral service.

The source of the fever, its true nature, and the number of deaths it caused will never be known. Histories and medical articles written later give varying accounts. George Sutherland wrote that "the *Jacmel Packet* arrived from Batavia carrying with her, a terrible fatal fever, known as *Yellow Jack*, which nearly decimated the small population and gave Burketown a very bad name. Of course there was no doctor, no medical aid and no proper food and the poisonous grog dispensed helped the heavy mortality". Another historian, E. Palmer, blamed the *Margaret and Mary*. He said she touched at some infected port in Java and on her arrival in Burketown a fatal sickness broke out. All hands on the ship died except the captain, whose wife fell a victim. A new crew had to be engaged before the vessel could leave the port. Palmer claimed that there was little doubt that the infection was traceable to this vessel. He added that there must have been at least a hundred besides those on the surrounding stations who died from the epidemic. The little cemetery soon looked like that of an old established town, so numerous were the graves. Shortly after this, Burketown was absolutely deserted. Not a living soul remained and nothing was left to mark the spot except heaps of empty bottles and jam tins. There were some large iron pots belonging to a boiling down works and stumps where once there had been buildings. The hulls of the *Gazelle* and the *Firefly* lay falling to pieces but no one was left to sigh over Burketown's fallen fortunes or say a dirge in memory of its history. Later, of course, people returned, and abandoned stations were once again taken up.

Medical writers have from time to time debated the cause of the epidemic. As there were no practitioners in the area at the time, they have to depend on lay descriptions of the disease. Yellow fever, as suggested by Sutherland's "Yellow Jack", has been summarily dismissed as a possibility. Two diseases — typhoid fever and malaria — have their supporters. One writer, Aitken White, believed that the fever was due to the typhoid organism, as some of the patients were said to have exhibited the typical rose spots of typhoid fever — scattered marks of that colour on their abdomen. There was no doctor to diagnose rashes in Burketown at the time, and, as pointed out by Philip James. these spots might have been caused by prickly heat so frequently experienced in hot climates. The *Port Denison Times* correspondent spoke of gastric symptoms suggestive of typhoid. But such symptoms occur in other diseases. John Elkington, Queensland's second commissioner of public health, and Ted Derrick, Queensland's famous medical researcher and discoverer of Q fever, selected malignant malaria as the culprit, an illness that has gastric symptoms. For years after the epidemic a diagnosis of "Gulf Fever" was given by medical practitioners and patients themselves to describe any sickness in which the temperature was raised.

POSTSCRIPT. The following paragraph appeared in the *Australian Medical Journal* for 1868.

> A correspondent of the Port Denison Times writing from Burketown, says two medical men who lately went there in the hope of making a fortune out of the large practice to be got from the constantly prevailing endemic fever have abandoned the profession and are now respectively keeping a public-house and tending a mob of "kanakas" whatever these last may be.

The Case of the Missing Head

About 10 a.m. on 6 November 1867, Mary Peterson, a domestic at the Bedford Arms, near the Mackenzie River, some 150 miles west of Rockhampton, went to the camp of the Clermont-Rockhampton gold escort a quarter of a mile away to ask for a billy can borrowed by the escort troopers the night before. When she was close to the camp, she saw one of the troopers lying on his back covered with a blanket. Mary called, but when he did not reply she thought he was asleep, and left without carrying out her errand. The escort was returning to Clermont after carrying gold from the Peak Downs gold mine to Rockhampton. It consisted of two troopers — John Power and Patrick Cahill — who had both been doing the job for three years. Thomas Griffin, the recently-appointed second gold commissioner at Rockhampton, had travelled with the men as far as the Bedford Arms at Mackenzie River. About 5 a.m. on the morning that Mary Peterson went to claim her billy can, Griffin had left the area with Alfred Bedford, the licensee of the Bedford Arms, to start on a journey arranged the preceding night. They planned to ride to Westwood, the terminus of the newly-constructed railway from Rockhampton and then catch the train to Rockhampton. Nothing further was heard from the escort camp on 6 November, but the next day John Peterson, Mary's husband, who was also employed at the hotel, made a startling discovery.

While searching for a guest's horse near the troopers' camp, he noticed one of them lying in the same position described by his wife the day before. Receiving no answer to his greeting of "Good-morning", he made a closer examination. Both men were dead. Peterson returned quickly to the hotel to give the alarm. A guest volunteered to ride to report the discovery to the native police station further down the Mackenzie River. Acting Sub-Inspector Richard Stokes left for the scene while his colleague, Lieutenant Uhr, rode to the railhead 100 miles away to relay the message to Inspector Elliott of the Rockhampton police. Elliott left for Mackenzie River, taking with him Detective Kilfedder. Griffin, who had arrived at Rockhampton with the publican

Bedford the day before the news was relayed to Inspector Elliott, volunteered to return with the party, an offer that was accepted. Later, the health officer for Rockhampton district, David Salmond, also set out for the scene. Before he left Rockhampton, Elliott interviewed Thomas Hall, the manager of the Australian Stock Bank, who told him that the escort had left Rockhampton carrying £8,000 in notes from the bank. Bedford's account of his journey from Mackenzie with Griffin was also part of the evidence collected by the police. On the way Inspector Elliott had several conversations with Griffin. The first press report of the occurrence appeared in the *Rockhampton Bulletin* on 9 November. It read:

> Intelligence of a dreadful case of poisoning near the Mackenzie River was received in town yesterday afternoon. The first news was brought to Westwood by Lieutenant Uhr, who despatched Constable Monahan, with a brief note to Rockhampton; the Constable arrived by train yesterday afternoon. He reports that troopers . . . Power and . . . Cahill, both young men, who had been about three years in the escort, were found dead in their camp, on Wednesday; it is conjectured from the effects of poison, as two pigs, which had eaten of a portion of the matter vomited by the deceased troopers, had died in consequence. The troopers were returning to Clermont, and had a quantity of money in their charge. Mr. Griffin arrived with the two troopers at the Mackenzie River on Tuesday night. The men had breakfast and dinner at the Bedford Arms, and a portion of two bottles of porter, and then returned to their camp, about a quarter of a mile from the hotel. Mr. Griffin, who spent a portion of the day at the hotel, also returned to the camp in the evening. He started for Rockhampton with Mr. Bedford, the landlord of the Bedford Arms, at a quarter to 5 on the following morning, arrived in Rockhampton by the half-past 5 train on Thursday. No definite particulars have been received as to the time when the bodies were discovered, or to whether the money was carried off. Being a return escort, no thought of any money being in their charge would occur to the minds of those discovering the bodies. If their deaths were the result of poisoning by parties intent on the money, its absence is easily accounted for. No mention is, however, made of the money in the report. Lieutenant Uhr rode 100 miles in ten hours with his arm in a sling, and sent on the Constable from Westwood.

Inspector Elliott and his party reached the death scene about 9 a.m. on 11 November. The bodies were exhumed from the shallow grave in which they had been buried and Dr Salmond found holes in each skull which were obviously made by bullets. The party searched for tracks around the campsite, and available witnesses were interviewed. Two hours later, Griffin, the new second gold commissioner, was arrested on suspicion of having murdered Power and Cahill.

Thomas John Augustus Griffin was born in County Antrim, Ireland, in 1832. After serving gallantly in the Crimean War he migrated to Australia in 1857. During the voyage, he befriended a widow of some means, whom he married shortly after their arrival in Melbourne. After squandering most of her money, he deserted to join the New South Wales Force. At the time of the Canoona gold rush, he was sent by the New South Wales Force to Rockhampton to take charge of the police force there. Later he went to Brisbane where he was appointed chief magistrate and gold commissioner at Clermont, the town established with the discovery of the Peak Downs goldfield. The *Brisbane Courier* said that while in these positions ''he seems to have had the usual luck of police magistrates in our small towns — making very admiring friends and very bitter enemies''. One who certainly did not admire him was Oscar de Satge, a prominent pastoralist and chief magistrate of Clermont. De Satge had started an enquiry after he discovered Griffin had stolen a letter which criticized his work. When the enquiry was held in Brisbane, few witnesses could attend, and Griffin was exonerated. Not long before the deaths of the troopers, Griffin was transferred as second gold commissioner to Rockhampton. It was reported that at a farewell function ''several of the speakers referred to the late contemptible attack upon Mr Griffin, and pointed out that many of the statements made were absolutely false, while others were perversions of the truth''. When he was transferred from Clermont, he was no longer in charge of the gold escort. In going with it back to Clermont, Griffin was acting outside his jurisdiction.

A preliminary enquiry was conducted at Mackenzie by bank inspector Abbott, who had gone to the scene of the crime and was the only justice of the peace available. A later hearing was conducted by W.H. Wiseman, the police magistrate at Rockhampton. The main point which made police suspect Griffin was that several of the bank notes in the bundles given to the escort were able to be traced because the numbers had been recorded by bank officers. Before leaving Clermont, Griffin had been entrusted with gold to the value of £252 by six Chinese. For several weeks he had been unable to settle when pressed by them. When they set off from Rockhampton, Griffin made several excuses for not going on with the journey. However, just prior to the final departure of the escort from Rockhampton after several of these false starts, he was suddenly able to pay the debt. Sergeant Julian, sacked by Griffin from the escort, during this time, recorded that the commissioner had charge of the money while other members were absent. As soon as the Chinese were paid, they went to the bank to change the notes into sovereigns, and the notes were recognized as part of the sum sent with the escort. Griffin paid for drinks with another note after he had returned to Rockhampton with Bedford. Yet a third was found in a spot where Griffin had left Bedford while riding to Westwood. The police surmised that Griffin had removed £252 from the escort money while it was in his possession before the troopers left Rockhampton, and stole the remainder after he had shot Power and Cahill. Further evidence on which the police relied was the conversation that Griffin had with Hall, the bank manager, when the first news arrived that the troopers had been poisoned. He said that poisoning would not have been the way the men had met their deaths. He felt sure that it would be found that they had been shot. This was rather a strange statement to make under the circumstances. Then he told Inspector Elliott three different versions of how he left the camp on the morning the men died. First he said that Power was on watch, then he stated that it was Cahill who was on duty, and later he claimed that both troopers were asleep.

At the end of the Rockhampton hearing, Wiseman remanded Griffin to the Rockhampton gaol, to await his trial for murder at the March 1868 sittings of the Rockhampton assizes. The charge was heard before Mr Justice Lutwyche and a jury of twelve. The attorney general, Ratcliffe Pring, QC, and Charles Lilley, QC, appeared for the Crown. After Griffin's original counsel, Gore Jones, died a few days before the trial date, he refused to apply for a postponement and accepted the offer of three junior members of the bar, led by Edward MacDevitt, to represent him. After the jury had listened to sixty witnesses give evidence which was wholly circumstantial it retired to consider the verdict. In an hour, the foreman announced a verdict of guilty. Given the opportunity, Griffin gave a long, disconnected speech in which he professed his innocence. The closing part of the trial was reported in the *Rockhampton Bulletin*:

> His Honour then said, Thomas Griffin, you have been found guilty by a jury of your countrymen, of the crime of wilful murder, and I can say that sitting in my place here I never heard circumstantial evidence of guilt more satisfactory, or more conclusive. I will add little that will give you more pain. My own feelings are deep and painful enough when I see you in your position [guilty] of a crime unparalleled in the

annals of Australian history. I am unequal to the task of expressing the pain, the anguish, and the horror I feel. I'll only do what the law compels me, that is to pass its sentence, and that is that you, Thomas John Griffin, be taken from the place where you stand to the place from whence you came, and there, at such time as may be appointed by the Acting-Governor, with the advice of the Executive Council, be hanged by the neck until you are dead; and may God, in His infinite mercy, have mercy on your soul. The venerable Judge was deeply affected at the conclusion of the address and was overcome with emotion, a feeling that communicated itself to many in the Court.

The *Brisbane Courier* greeted the verdict with an editorial.

In the records of crime in these colonies there are many blood-ensanguined pages, but taking into consideration all the terrible details, there, perhaps, will be found none of more abhorrent hue than those which chronicle the Mackenzie murders. A jury of Griffin's peers have pronounced him guilty of the blood of Cahill and Power, and if they are right, his crime stands out from almost all others that we know of, in horrible relief. If he murdered these men he did [so] to cover the plunder of money entrusted to them and regarded from no other point than this, the deed would sink into the ordinary category of the many atrocious crimes in which human life has been sacrificed to greed. But in this particular instance the infamy of the act is aggravated a thousand-fold by the fact that the men whom Griffin slew were his comrades in a dangerous service — his own friends. It is the treachery of the deed that most appals one. In the most imminent perils which might befall them, these men had a right to reckon on the aid and defence of one who, in the characters of friend, comrade, and superior officer was triply bound to them. That he could coolly plot and plan the death of these men, and slay in their sleep those whom every sentiment of honour and manliness bound him to protect even at hazard of his own life, is hardly to be realised; but that he did so, twelve men, hearing the whole evidence without fear or favour, have on their oaths declared that they believe.

An appeal against the sentence was heard by the chief justice, James Cockle, and Judge Lutwyche, sitting as a superior court. It relied largely upon a question put by the judge in his summing up, "If Griffin did not commit the murder, who did?" It was contended that it was not for the jury to assume that Griffin must have committed the murder, but for the Crown to prove that he did commit it. In dismissing the appeal, the chief justice said that "A Judge's summing up must not be regarded as consisting of a set of separate sentences, but must be taken as a whole. The part which had been objected to in the present case might, under one aspect, appear a very strong way of putting the matter to the jury; but yet, if the whole were considered, it might be the very best way of putting to the jury the true point that they had to decide".

Griffin was hanged at the Rockhampton gaol on 1 June 1868. He spent most of the night before with Rev. Mr Smith, a Presbyterian minister whose efforts to induce Griffin to confess his guilt were in vain. The principal turnkey, John Lee, joined the minister in the attempt to overcome the convicted man's obduracy. He died as most who knew him believed he would, denying his guilt and showing great nerve and firmness to the last. When all preparations were made and Griffin waited on the scaffold for the final act, the hangman asked if he had anything to confess. Griffin replied in a firm voice, "No, I have nothing to confess". The body was cut down after thirty-five minutes. Four doctors pronounced life extinct: David Salmond, Archibald Robertson, William Callaghan and Guido Thon. Griffin was buried in the Rockhampton cemetery. The *Rockhampton Bulletin* editorial described the execution in picturesque language, and then voiced an opinion on capital punishment.

> In the discharge of a sad and painful duty, we witnessed yesterday morning the killing of a human being by the minister of human justice — the public hangman. The scene was pitiful, brutal, and revolting, and the shuddering crowd, who gazed on the doomed man as he stood on the fatal drop with the hideous night-cap drawn over his face, felt their hearts throb with pity and sympathy for the victim of his own ungovernable passions hurried away in the flush and pride of his manhood from the bright sunlight to the dark cold grave.
>
> If Griffin had been condemned to perpetual and solitary confinement, where, cut off from the old associations and the society whose applause he so much coveted, he would have had ample time for reflection on his horrible crime, and there might be some hope that he would at last repent. He might also have been induced in the course of time to disclose the place where he had planted the bank notes, which are now lost, probably to the bank. Perpetual imprisonment might fall short in its terrors of the swift justice of the gallows. On the brutal minds of the class predisposed by ignorance and want to crime, the gallows may have its influence, especially when capital punishment is inflicted within the walls of a gaol, and surrounded by all the gloomy accessories of the law and where the hoarse plaudits of a brutalised mob to die game, are shut out from the dying wretch's ears. But there is a higher class of criminal, of which Griffin is a type, to whom death by hanging, sudden and painless, generally would be preferable to a life-long punishment. They don't mind hanging and ninetenths of the educated murderers face their deaths calmly and firmly. Opinion has fluctuated a good deal on this subject.

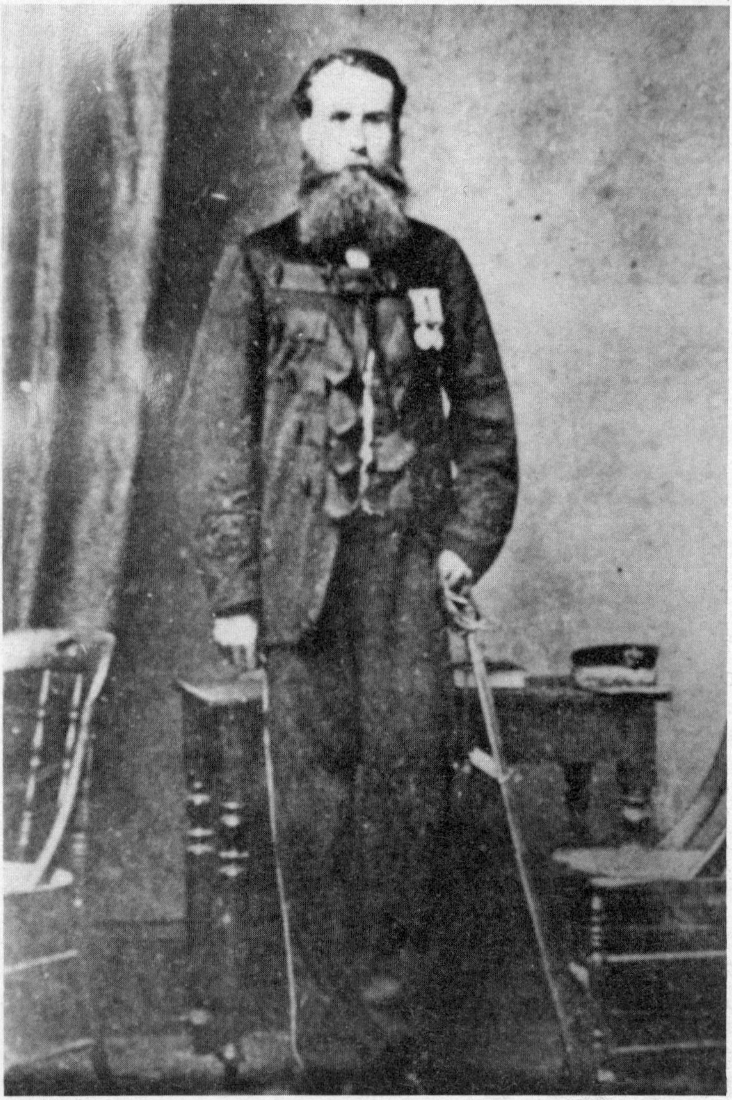

Thomas Griffin (around 1865), hanged for the murder of two gold escorts. (Courtesy Oxley Library)

Whilst society exists as at present, murderers will, we suppose, be removed from the world as quickly as possible. In young countries, where crime is prevalent, and the law is but little respected, there is but little room for the exercise of a mercy fitted for a higher and purer civilisation. We may wish for a change, yet not hope to see it in our day. If there will be murderers, there must be hangmen; and our creed must still be "blood for blood".

The newspaper's surmise that the stolen money might be lost for good was astray, and the general opinion that Griffin had not confessed was not quite the case. On the day after the execution, Alfred Grant, assistant turnkey at the gaol, reported to the sheriff that Griffin had secretly confessed to him some days before he was hanged. The convicted man had promised to tell where the money was hidden in return for help in an escape attempt. If the plan failed, Griffin was to be supplied with a knife or poison to allow him to commit suicide. When Grant convinced the prisoner that these plans were impracticable, the prisoner then said he would reveal the whereabouts of the money if Grant would promise to send £500 to Griffin's sister in Ireland. Grant confided in the principal turnkey, John Lee. On three occasions, the turnkeys went to an area not far from Rockhampton, using plans drawn by Griffin, but they failed to find the money. When this information was made public, there was much speculation on why the turnkeys had not reported the confession till after the execution. Did they believe that Griffin was lying when they failed to find the booty? Did they decide not to risk handling easily traceable notes and seek the reward of £200 being offered by the bank? Why did not Lee tell Rev. Smith about the confession, to help him convince Griffin to confess publicly? When the news got out, Lee went with the police, the sheriff and Hall, the bank manager who had given evidence that Griffin had told him the troopers would be found to have been shot, not poisoned. Using the plans that Griffin had given the turnkeys, Lee went almost immediately to a hollow tree stump and recovered a valise containing the money. He denied strongly that he had known its location before. The bank paid the turnkeys the reward, but when the colonial secretary considered the report of an enquiry by Wiseman, the police magistrate, into the withholding of the information, the turnkeys were both dismissed.

But that was not to be the end of the case. On the day of Griffin's burial, the sexton told the chairman of the cemetery trustees that he had heard that an attempt would be made to take Griffin's body from the grave. This information was not passed on to the police, but the sexton was instructed to keep as close a watch as possible. For most of the week he watched for part of the night. About 7 p.m. on the second night, the body of a man who had died on a ship in port was brought for burial without ceremony. The sexton buried him in Griffin's grave. Six days after the first burial, the sexton reported that the grave had been disturbed. An imprint which could have been made by a coffin was easily visible next to the grave. Clots of hair, some pieces of skin of human appearance and something like brains were found nearby. At the foot of the grave was a bottle containing carbolic acid. The sexton sounded the grave with a rod and touched a coffin much closer to the surface than that at which he had buried the second body. Later, a sheath knife was discovered about five metres away. Approval by telegraph to exhume the bodies was obtained from the colonial secretary. The grave was opened in the presence of cemetery and police officers and Doctors Salmond and Thon. As estimated by the sexton, one coffin was found at a higher level than he had buried it. The lid had been removed and loosely refastened. The body was unmolested. Further removal of soil revealed a second coffin also closer to the surface than Griffin had been buried. Again, there were evidence of interference with the coffin. The lid was easily removed. One horrified look was enough. There was only a headless trunk. The head was gone. The body was identified as Griffin by two doctors who had been present at the hanging. Decapitation would have been easily carried out with a knife, as the doctors had previously dissected the back of the neck after the execution. A government reward of £20 was offered for any information leading to the identification and apprehension of the offenders. There was severe criticism by many who thought that the amount offered was too paltry. Two rival newspapers in Rockhampton vied with each other in their efforts to describe these new developments. The *Northern Argus*, in dramatic fashion, reported that:

> The hand that did the ruthless deed was there, and when the body was rolled out, a piece of paper fell with it, on which was yet to be seen the tracing of what had once been a flower — the gift of one loving and loved — but the head that planned, plotted, and guided, was not there — it had been severed from the trunk — an easy task, for the work had been already half done by the doctor in the gaol after the execution, and was borne away to gratify the hunger of science or gold. It is on its way to grace the studio of the surgeon, to form a portion of the attractions of a show, or to have features of wax moulded over the skull, and exhibited in a chamber of horrors to satisfy the mania of the never satiated curiosity of the million. The body was decomposed and swollen, and presented a most disgusting and never-to-be-forgotten picture — a picture which never ought to have been commissioned, but which was called into life in all its fearful and naked horrors, by carelessness, want of proper feeling, and an utter disregard of those finer touches of propriety and kindly sentiment which are, thank Heaven, still existent, and we believe and hope, deathless in the human bosom.

Part of the *Rockhampton Bulletin*'s effort was:

> Twenty pounds for Griffin's head! Such is the magnificent reward our moral Government offer for the discovery of the perpetrators of a gross outrage. Why, any proprietor of a Chamber of Horrors would think it cheap at £50 and would think nothing of giving £30 as hush-money to persons engaged in the outrage. We hold that it makes not the slightest difference whether it was the head of a saint or a sinner that was robbed from the grave. The murderer — Griffin — had as much right to his narrow grave, once laid in it as My Lord Bishop or the Lord Mayor of London to his family vault. The desecration of the dead is a barbarity which this age will not tolerate, and it is a disgrace to the Government that the reward they offer for the detection of the crime is not more than they would offer for a good horse or a bullock. We hope the police will use proper vigilance; we know that they are in possession of information which points indubitably to two persons, and we expect that they will do their duty for Griffin when dead as they did against him when living.

Despite the many rumours and the supposition that the police had two suspects, no arrests were made. Weeks, months and then years passed and the mystery remained unsolved. In 1904, Bird included a chapter on the MacKenzie murders in his *History of Early Rockhampton*: "After a lapse of 36 years there can be no harm in saying that there were only two men implicated in the removal of Griffin's head. The two are still residents of Rockhampton and one of them has Griffin's skull yet." The publication brought no public identification of the grave robbers. But in June 1922, the Melbourne *Australasian* published this article:

> THE MURDERER'S HEAD
>
> By D
>
> There were three of them; three staid, sober, grave gentlemen, and they wanted Griffin's head — Griffin, the Queensland Gold Commissioner who was hanged for the cold-blooded murder of his two troopers. Griffin had been buried that morning, and three friends — banker, surgeon and editor — foregathered in the surgery to discuss what the skull of such a callous murderer would be like.
>
> "I'd like to examine it," said the surgeon.
>
> "What about getting it, then, and studying at leisure?" said the editor, who was Irish.
>
> "Ye gods! What a suggestion!" remarked the tall, slim banker, as he raised his long form and began striding up and down the spacious room.
>
> Not one of the three gave a moment's thought to the professional ruin that might follow discovery. Plot after plot was enthusiastically

advanced by one and the other, and the three clever heads set themselves to the formation of a plan. No one but themselves was to be let into the adventure, no help hired, no one trusted in any way.

Finally the following plan was carried out successfully. The three conspirators left their separate residences quietly after dark, the tall banker carrying a spade hidden under his dark overcoat; the surgeon carried the necessary instruments for decapitation and the bag for the head. The editor, like a true Irish conspirator, had his dark lantern "handy". Taking a roundabout way, they met at the graveside. (The official position of one of them rendered access easy.) The lantern door was opened, and the banker unfastened the spade which he had tied close to his body, and, after vigorous digging, the soft earth was soon displaced. Then the surgeon's task began, and deftly his part was gone through, the editor shining his light on the bottom of the grave. The head was soon severed — not neatly — and placed in the bag. The banker resumed his spade work and quickly filled in the grave, smoothing and arranging as it had been before opening. The lantern was closed, and the conspirators separated, each returning by another roundabout route to his own premises. A bath and a change of clothes and three decorous gentlemen met as usual for evening whist at the surgeon's residence.

The surgeon in the meantime had examined the head, written down his observations, and had placed it in chemicals to remove the fleshy parts. The examination of the skull provided interest for a whole night. As the three cronies had been accustomed to see the early dawn in at times when leaving each other's house, the banker and the editor wended their happy way together to their respective homes, the former carrying the skull, wrapped in brown paper, also the spade, attached to his back by a thin rope. The skull was at once placed in the bank safe.

Yet, for all the precautions taken, the disturbance of the grave was noticed, and it was opened by the authorities, and the decapitation discovered. The surgeon was called in. He said the beheading was performed evidently by a clumsy person; the editor was requested to insert advertisements in his paper offering a reward of £10 for information leading to the conviction of the offender. Banker, surgeon and editor discussed the affair with all and sundry and listened to theories and became enthusiastic over clues, but not a breath of suspicion was attached to the principals, and after several insertions the advertisements and reward were withdrawn and the incident passed into the limbo of forgotten things.

When very young I heard the story from two of the principals, the editor and the banker, and many years after the incident was the skull displayed under a glass in the banker's drawing-room.

The pen that wrote the article in the *Australasian* belonged to Daisy Bates, who relied on journalism as a source of income while she lived and worked among the Australian Aborigines. Elizabeth Salter, in her biography of Daisy Bates published in 1972, identified the three conspirators as R.H. White (banker), Thadeus O'Kane (editor) and O'Callaghan (surgeon). Biographies of White and O'Kane indicate grave-robbing was a likely activity in which they would be involved. As a young officer in the Bank of New South Wales at Deniliquin, Robert Hoddle White once pursued some bushrangers who had robbed the bank. He recovered some of the money and was instrumental in having the leader arrested. He was appointed manager of the Rockhampton branch of the bank in 1864. He won rewards for his defence against five armed men at the Currie Hotel on the Gympie fields in April 1868. About the same time, he was involved in a dispute with junior officers of the Rockhampton company of the Queensland Volunteer Rifles of which he was the captain. During this he was challenged to a duel by the company's surgeon, Archibald Robertson, who was present at Griffin's hanging. Thadeus O'Kane was a sub-editor of the *Rockhampton Bulletin* at the time of Griffin's hanging. He was described as "one of the most colourful, influential and hard-hitting figures in early Queensland journalism; he lost count of the libel actions he faced". In his own words he had "a warm temperament and strong passion, and was a staunch friend and a bitter enemy".

William Callaghan's history does not suggest that grave-robbing was an activity in which he was likely to have been involved. A graduate of the College of Surgeons, London, he was registered as a medical practitioner in Queensland in 1861, being number six on the first register of the colony's newly appointed medical board. He went to Rockhampton where he replaced Robertson at the public hospital, with which he was associated for the next half-century. Besides becoming one of the town's best-known doctors, he was prominent in public affairs generally. The naming of the racecourse, Callaghan Park, in his honour reflected his great love of horses, his breeding of thoroughbreds and his interest in racing. If he did take part in the grave-robbing, it could be surmised that he wished to use Griffin's head to test the theory of phrenology which was current at the time. The basis of this pseudo-science was first put forward by German physician Franz Josef Gall early in the nineteenth century. Gall quite correctly suggested that different parts of the brain were involved with different parts of the body. He suggested a correlation between the shape of the brain and emotional and temperamental characteristics. Taking his theory further, he submitted that the shape of the brain could, in turn, be deduced from any superficial unevenness of the skull. Thus there arose the belief that a man's character could be determined by the bumps on his head.

Lorna McDonald, in her book *Rockhampton — A History of the City and District*, published in 1981, states that many were aware that Dr Callaghan was the ringleader in the grave-robbing, and the skull remained in his possession. The same writer also raises the interesting possibility that Griffin suffered from a mental illness. She draws attention to a letter written in England in 1918 by W.H. Leighton Bailey. Bailey claims that he reported the Griffin case for the *Northern Argus* and that he was present when Griffin's head was taken. The former report said that, had Dr Callaghan studied Griffin's mental state while he was alive as carefully as he had used his skull, he might have had compassion for a sick man. Griffin's history certainly suggests some degree of instability, but from the records it is difficult to estimate the extent. During the first hearing, Sergeant Julian said that he had had a conversation with the troopers on the way from Roobottom's, before the escort left Rockhampton, pointing to Griffin's state of mind. He considered that Griffin was mad then, and he thought he was still mad. Of course this evidence was given after Griffin had sacked Julian. Sub-Inspector Balfrey, of Clermont, who had known Griffin for seven years, said that the gold commissioner was not eccentric. Griffin was under treatment by Dr Benson in Clermont, but the illness seems to have been a physical one — intermittent fever. In the trial before Judge Lutwyche, Griffin's counsel did not raise the question of any illness. It is unlikely that a plea of not guilty on the grounds of insanity was considered for submission by his defending barristers.

It is not surprising that there are discrepancies between the various accounts. Bird and Lorna McDonald suggest that the skull stayed in Rockhampton. Daisy Bates said that she was shown the skull by White. As she did not to come to Australia until 1884, and White had left Rockhampton long before this, she must have seen it in New South Wales, if her story is true. Her account also says Callaghan was called by the police when the head was taken and the doctor reported that the work was that of a clumsy person. Perhaps this is an embellishment in an otherwise true story. More likely the true story will never be known.

Snakes in the Asylum

When Queensland built its first mental hospital, three doctors applied to run it: a liar, a cheat, and a medico who had once been certified deranged. The three were politely refused. But the doctor who did get the job was eventually dismissed when it was revealed patients were locked naked in cells with only straw to sleep on, or died without anyone noticing or caring. The hospital had a stormy beginning.

After Queensland became a separate colony, but before the mental hospital was built, lunatics, as they were called, were held in the gaol and usually mixed freely with the criminals there. They were not welcome at the public hospital. Hugh Bell, the hospital's medical superintendent in 1854, wrote this note about a mental patient: "So violent, I was obliged to put on the strait jacket — removed to gaol". Occasionally, the justices committed a patient to the hospital instead of the gaol. This happened in 1857 and immediately the hospital committee secretary wrote to the magistrates bench advising that the hospital had no facilities to care for such patients. Before 1859, the gaol to which mental patients were sent was the old female factory in Queen Street, where later the General Post Office was built.

When Moreton Bay separated from New South Wales to become the colony of Queensland, the first governor, Sir George Ferguson Bowen, wrote to Sir William Denison, governor of New South Wales, requesting that the arrangement of transferring lunatics to the Tarban Creek Lunatic Asylum, Sydney, continue. The request fell on deaf ears. There was now only one place in which such patients could be accommodated — the gaol. By this time, a new gaol had been built at Petrie Terrace to hold 144 prisoners.

At first the gaol accommodation was quite sufficient to meet the demands. In January 1861, the returns from the gaoler, Samuel Sneyd, showed that the inmates totalled 54, of whom 8 were lunatics. However, the numbers increased rapidly. By July 1863, Sheriff William Brown advised the colonial secretary that there were 181 prisoners and lunatics. He was compelled to place 24 men in the lower floor of the women's ward at night and 33 men slept in the schoolroom, the dimensions of which were forty-six feet long by twenty feet wide. In addition to this overcrowding, a visiting justice, Buttanshaw, pointed out another inconvenience. The pump which supplied water was situated in the women's ward. This necessitated male prisoners spending considerable time each day in the women's ward. Buttanshaw added that "in the case of female lunatics it is often difficult to get them to wear even the slightest covering and under the circumstances alluded to, discipline in the ward cannot be caried out". The overcrowding prevented any classification or segregation in the prison, so criminals and lunatics mixed freely. Darvall, another visiting justice, reported the lack of shelter in the exercise yard where the inmates spent many day hours, even in the heat of summer:

> There is an open shed with no sides to it and which affords very slight shelter. To obtain that you have to move your seat as the sun goes round. The reflection from the stone seats is intolerable. Some who have been confined for some time are absolutely black. You can hardly know them from the natives of the colony.

The government of the young colony was aware of the problems at the gaol and in 1862, building started on a lunatic asylum some twelve miles from Brisbane, where the Brisbane River joins Woogaroo Creek. A temporary asylum using other premises was also considered. Charles Tiffin, the colonial architect, William Brown, the sheriff and Kearsey Cannan, the visiting medical officer to the gaol, were sent to inspect premises belonging to Mr Franz at German Station, now Nundah. They reported that with some alterations the various buildings would be suitable to accommodate the mental patients, but no action was taken on their recommendation.

While the asylum was being built, the government received applications from three doctors for the position of superintendent. They came from William Ewington, Jacob Swift and Jonathan Labatt. It is not surprising that all three were rejected. Ewington forwarded his application to Government Bowen, as he believed that it was only by "addressing the Governor in Chief of Queensland that any important appointment could be made". He claimed that he was known to the Marquis of Breadalbane, the Earl of Winterton and the brother of Lord Clarina, Elm Park, Limerick. Ewington felt certain that all these names would at least be familiar to His Excellency. Attached to Ewington's file is a letter from the immigration agent stating there could be no doubt whatever that Mr Ewington was guilty of a most deliberate and heartless act of swindling in connection with £46 which had been advanced to him in England. The agent requested every help in prosecuting the doctor. Manning, the principal undersecretary, advised Ewington that the government was unable to confer on him the appointment he sought. He was saved from prosecution by paying the money.

The second applicant, Jacob Meade Swift, was a colourful character. After coming to Moreton Bay early in 1851, he quickly secured important positions in a settlement which had few doctors. Within a few months, he was appointed health officer for the port of Brisbane, visiting surgeon to the Brisbane Hospital, and coroner. Apparently not satisfied with the income from these positions and his private practice, he thought up a scheme to further augment his bank account. At this time, gold had just been discovered in southern parts of Australia. The citizens of Moreton Bay, envious of what they considered to be the good fortune of the southerners, quickly promised a reward to the first person to discover the precious metal in Moreton Bay. The amount promised the lucky discoverer soon passed £900 — no mean sum in 1851. Swift reported to the reward committee that he had discovered gold in River Terrace, South Brisbane, and produced a nugget to support his claim. J.J. Knight, in his book *In the Early Days*, tells what followed next:

> Some cracked stones; others delved holes. While reinforcements with shovels, hammers, crowbars, and such implements could be seen travelling through South Brisbane. One party had a prospecting pan; another a colander. One had a legitimate cradle in which was stowed away the necessary bedding for camping out and the same provident party also carried a bucket of water for washing the sand. Of course the field turned out to be a duffer, but no one would believe this until Dr Swift's application for reward came up before the committee for consideration and there was an unexplained absence of both the doctor and the exhibit.

Dr Swift's application to manage the Woogaroo Asylum was refused.

The third applicant, Jonathan Labatt, at least had some experience with lunatic asylums. He had been imprisoned for a month as a lunatic, and was seeking compensation from the government for wrongful incarceration. Swift and Labatt were advised that it was the intention of the government to procure a professional gentleman who had more recently been connected with lunatic establishments in England. When the asylum was ready for occupation, no professional gentleman from England appeared, and the position was given to Kearsey Cannan, who had been visiting surgeon to the gaol since 1850, and to the lunatics there from 1864.

Arriving in Moreton Bay in 1843, Cannan was the first private medical practitioner in Brisbane. He was amiable and tolerant, but a lax administrator. The lunatics were moved from the gaol to Woogaroo on 10 January 1865. Sheriff Halloran advised the colonial secretary that the "whole of the lunatics under confinement in Her Majesty's Gaol at Brisbane, 57 males and 12 females, were safely placed on board the steamer, *Settler*, at half past eight in the morning". In turn, Cannan reported that no one had fallen overboard; all arrived safely and were comfortably housed. The main building was a two-storeyed brick structure. The top storey contained eight wards for 100 male patients. Downstairs, the female patients slept in four wards with accommodation for 54 inmates. Separate buildings provided a kitchen and office facilities.

Almost from its inception, the Woogaroo Asylum was the subject of several enquiries. It was one of the institutions examined by a select committee of the Legislative Assembly appointed in 1866 to enquire into the hospitals of the colony. During his evidence before this committee, Cannan said that "the principal medical comfort allowed is beer. The men who go out to work varies from eighteen to twenty and there are about eight females who work in the laundry and get a glass of beer daily. I give them this extra, because I consider it good for bodily health, and I believe that good bodily health is essential to recovery from mental illness. I believe it is a great part of the cure to nourish patients well". The committee was favourably impressed and said that Dr Cannan appeared eminently qualified for the duties of his office, and, doubtless much of the success of the institution and its high state of efficiency were due to his skill and energy.

Not long after this, Patrick Barry, a warder, "laid an accusation of a very serious character against the chief warder, William Haddon, viz., that the chief warder 'had to do' with one of the female patients". Lieutenant Colonel Gray, police magistrate at Ipswich, conducted an enquiry and found that both the chief warder and the patient had been missing for two hours. He concluded that the only reasonable assumption under such circumstances was that they were together for immoral purposes. The chief warder was dismissed. However, Barry, who had made the complaint, was suspended also, because he had claimed that he had seen the two together when, in fact, he had heard about the episode from someone else.

Despite the glowing account of Cannan given by the select committee, the government was obviously worried about affairs at the asylum. In 1867, another committee was appointed to enquire into "the general management and working of the Lunatic Asylum at Woogaroo with a view to testing the efficiency of several officers connected with the institution and the means adopted by the surgeon superintendent for the security and proper treatment of the patients under his charge". Henry Challinor and Charles Coxen, members of the Legislative Assembly, and Hugh Massie, police magistrate, were asked to conduct the enquiry. Challinor, a medical practitioner, was asked to chair the committee, which he did for a number of meetings. He later withdrew and Coxen and Massie reported that they saw "no reason to believe that the present management of the Asylum was otherwise than of a satisfactory nature".

Still Cannan was not left in peace. In the summer of 1868–69 letters criticizing the asylum appeared in the Ipswich newspaper, *Queensland Times*, under pseudonyms. In a footnote the editor said that he had refused to publish a similar letter previously, but as scarcely a day passed that he did not hear rumours or information, proving an enquiry was necessary, he would not be doing his duty if he closed his columns to such statements. The writers of the anonymous letters were a dismissed warder and an ex-patient, both of whom, no doubt, bore a grudge against the institution. Under the pseudonym H.K., one said that "certainly anything more disgraceful than the state of the institution at the present time cannot be pointed out in any civilised or uncivilised country in the world . . . Sunstroke is the cause of perhaps sixty percent, of cases sent to the Asylum and were these patients treated rationally with kindness and a soothing application to the head, such as would be done at an hospital, they would recover rapidly: but then the doctor would lose his fee, the country saved a vast amount of expense and the patients a large amount of suffering. . . With regards to the visits of clergymen the place seems strangely neglected".

Another writer, De Facto, said:

> The Government could never have been aware of the method of conducting the department in question. Otherwise, they would never have allowed the disgraceful scenes which have taken place to go un-

> punished. It is astonishing, too, how persons such as Government officials and others, who occasionally visit the place, could be so deceived; but it is plain enough. They are generally shown around the premises by the surgeon or the chief warder; they see all is correct as they suppose, at least as far as outward appearance goes; but the treatment of the poor patients or the internal management of the place they never dream of; or that within those walls some poor fellows as sane as themselves were illegally detained, for want of proper medical attendance, an encumbrance to the public and five chances to one the prospect of a premature grave.

The letters appear vindictive and the statements exaggerated. However, like the editor of the *Queensland Times*, the government believed that an enquiry was necessary. A civil service commission of Patrick MacArthur, police magistrate, and A.M. Hutchinson, sub-collector of customs, was appointed for the task. Numerous witnesses both inside and outside the institution were examined. The writers of the letters to the press; the surgeon superintendent, Cannan, the warders and nurses; visiting justices, clergymen, and citizens whom Cannan requested on his behalf, gave evidence. The commission's report gives the appearance that its civil service authors, believing that their colleagues were guilty, endeavoured to paint as bright a picture as possible. An extract reads:

> Isolated and apart from incidental circumstances, the concurrent testimony of several witnesses would in some instances, seem to prove, to say the least, reprehensible harshness on the part of the surgeon superintendent. Viewed, however, in connection with the possible exigencies of each case, and the absence of means and appliances for better or milder treatment, the wilful character of the apparent harshness becomes doubtful and the possibility of its being more or less unavoidable under past and even present circumstances, suggest itself. For example, in the case of McCormack, the unfortunate man is represented as having been frequently locked up at night in a bare boarded cell, cold and comfortless, without clothes, and with no other bedding than loose straw. Now, per se, this must be regarded as harsh in the extreme, in fact, wilful cruelty, if needless. But, in the case specified, as in every other treated in like manner, it would seem the patients were afflicted with mania for destroying their clothes and bedding, so that for all practical purposes of warmth or decency they might possibly have been as well without. We do not pretend for a moment, excuse, much less justify such a mode of treatment; but in knowledge of the fact that want of padded cells, and the numerous humane expedients available in well equipped institutions to meet such cases, are wholly wanting here, the question has forced

Kearsey Cannan in 1871. The first superintendent of Woogaroo Asylum (now Wolston Park Hospital), he was plagued by controversy and faced several government enquiries into his treatment of the mentally ill. (Courtesy AMA Queensland branch)

> itself on our attention, and we leave it to your decision, — who is responsible — the Surgeon Superintendent or the Responsible Ministers who from time to time have charge of the department?. . .
>
> We may say generally, that regard having been had to the quality and conflict of the evidence, the allegations against the Surgeon Superintendent and the chief warder have failed of substantiation.

Having signed the above report as co-author, Hutchinson strangely submitted a separate and in parts conflicting report. In it he said:

> The least that can be said is that the buildings require to be remodelled, the establishment to be reorganised and the administration to be radically reformed. . . Whether the Surgeon Superintendent is or has been equal to the requirements of his position is a question I am neither competent nor called upon to decide.

The government concluded that despite the vindictiveness of the letters that started the enquiry, the evidence pointed to gross mismanagement. There was only one answer to the question of who was to blame — the surgeon superintendent or the responsible ministers. Dr Cannan would be responsible and must be dismissed. However, to find what was really necessary at Woogaroo, still another enquiry must be instigated. While debating the proposal to appoint a select committee from both houses of parliament, members referred to the report of the enquiry into the civil service.

The views of Mr Groom (Drayton and Toowoomba) were reported in the Queensland Parliamentary Debates:

> He was very much inclined to think, after reading the voluminous evidence taken by the commission appointed by the Government to inquire into the state of the asylum, that facts had been elicited which were sufficient to justify the Government in dismissing the whole of the officers connected with it. He thought if honourable members who had read all the horrors revealed to the British public during a number of years and all the tortures perpetrated in private asylums — accounts which they had probably at first looked upon as fiction, but had afterwards been obliged to realise as truth — would only compare them and place them side by side, with the horrible state of things brought to light by the commissioners at Woogaroo, they must come to the conclusion that a serious reflection had been cast on the colony. . .
>
> The evidence showed, that in the morning eighty or one hundred persons had been turned out into a yard and washed with the very mops with which the floors were scrubbed and that there was not even bedding for the poor creatures to lie upon — not even such common necessaries as were provided in every civilised country.

Mr Thompson (Ipswich) stated that:

> The charges comprised general neglect, particular neglect in particular cases, peculation, cruelty, drunkenness, and other immoralities and indecencies of all sorts . . . It appeared that some of the poor creatures who were inmates of the asylum, had been actually left to die with the blazing sun shining on their faces in this hot climate, it being doubtful whether the surgeon superintendent saw them either before or after they died.

Mr Walsh (Maryborough) joined the condemnation:

> The evidence showed that unfortunate inmates of this asylum, who were literally dying, had been treated like wild beasts: the very dogs, the sheep and the cattle in the colony were treated like princes in comparison with them.

Dr O'Doherty (North Brisbane) was the only member to say a word for his colleague. He endeavoured to excuse Cannan by claiming that the superintendent was hampered in his duties by the failure of the colonial secretary's department to supply requisitions from the asylum. Included in O'Doherty's speech was the following:

> During a visit to the asylum, he came across an unfortunate patient suffering in the last stages of dysentery — scarcely any life left in him. There was a case in which medicine and medical aid were required to save life. The only medicine that would have benefitted him was good port wine. He (Dr O'Doherty) asked the surgeon-superintendent how much wine was given to the patient daily. "My dear sir," said the doctor, "I have not been allowed to have wine in the place for the patients. Medical comforts are not allowed; they were stopped long since; and the only medical comforts I am allowed is vinegar."

The colonial secretary, Hodgson, speaking at the end of the debate, disagreed with O'Doherty and pointed to the evidence of Cannan before the enquiry into the hospitals of the colony when he said that he gave beer to the patients. He added:

> The Government had decided upon dispensing with the services of Dr Cannan. It gave him a great deal of pain to make such a statement. He had known Dr Cannan for the last twenty-seven years, and believed him to be a most amiable man, and one of the cleverest surgeons that ever came to the colonies. But the evidence they had before them showed that, at all events, he was scarcely the right man in the right place, at the asylum.

The *Brisbane Courier* supported the government's action in an editorial which began:

> The appointment of a joint-committee by both Houses of the Legislatures to inquire the state of the Woogaroo Lunatic Asylum is, we trust, the real commencement of a thorough and sweeping reform in the management of that institution. It is high time for something to be done in the matter, for it is impossible to imagine a more sickening recital than that of the evidence taken before the Commission recently appointed to inquire into the subject. The correspondence which appeared in the newspapers and led to the appointment of the Commission gave, after all, but a faint idea of the sufferings endured by the unfortunate patients from negative cruelty and positive neglect; and it is necessary to turn to the accounts of Bedlam as it existed 150 years ago, to meet a parallel to it. Even old Bedlam when at its worst was better, in some respects than Woogaroo is proved to have been up to within the last few weeks.

Cannan's dismissal on 19 May 1869 did not affect him professionally, nor did it greatly reduce the esteem in which he was held in the colony. He resumed his practice in Brisbane and his association with the Brisbane Hospital. Later he was appointed president of the medical board and a member of the Central Board of Health. The profession elected him president of the first Queensland Medical Society.

Shortly before his dismissal, Cannan had suffered from dysentery and was unable to attend to his work. He had asked for a locum tenens and the colonial secretary had immediately sent a telegram to Henry Challinor in Ipswich. Challinor had responded to the call, leaving a busy private practice to do so. When Cannan recovered, the relieving doctor had returned to Ipswich. Hearing the government's intentions to dismiss Cannan, Challinor offered his services to fill the vacancy. The government was delighted to accept his offer and the Ipswich doctor took over the reins two days after Cannan left. The two doctors were quite dissimilar. Challinor had reached Moreton Bay as the surgeon superintendent of the *Fortitude*, the first of Dr Dunmore Lang's immigrant ships to come to Moreton Bay in 1849. By the time he went to Woogaroo he had been in practice in Ipswich for twenty years. In that time he built up a reputation as a sound practitioner. He was a pillar of the Congregational Church and had a strong conscience, never afraid to voice his opinion. He entered parliament in 1861, and, speaking of his attitude in parliament, the *Moreton Bay Courier* said that "Challinor will stick to his own opinion on any question, in contemptuous defiance of the squatting majority". He was the type of man who would believe that it was his duty to leave his private practice and help the government clean up the administrative mess at the asylum. The new superintendent found that the records kept by his predecessor were meagre, and he wrote to Norton Manning, the respected superintendent of Tarban Creek (now Gladesville) Asylum in Sydney for advice on managing such an institution. From then on the official records and the statistical tables at Woogaroo were meticulously kept and full of information. Land was enclosed for recreational purposes, and amusements such as dancing, singing and music introduced. Sanitation was improved by substituting earth closets for the previous abominable privies, and ablution facilities brought to a reasonable standard. Challinor created a reputation for the institution that it so badly needed. He welcomed visitors to the asylum, but not the type which were the subject of a letter he wrote to the colonial secretary:

I do my self the honour to inform you that this place is very much infected with snakes, so much so that several have been killed in and about both branches of the Asylum and my residence. Not long since two were killed at short intervals in one of the female sleeping wards, two in the laundry, two or three near the chief nurse's cottage, another in one of the mens' dayrooms, two in the water closets, one in the gateway, several in the roadway between the two branches of the Asylum, not to mention several in the grounds. One evening, my servant trod on one coming from the kitchen to the house, and I think it was the next night I saw a brown one peering over my wife's shoulder, it having climbed up the back of the rocking chair on which she was seated. One had been killed not long before under the kitchen my children were accustomed to play in the heat of the day, and some have been killed in the garden close to the house. Most of them have been of a deadly kind and of a large size — some of them six feet long. I shall therefore be glad to receive the necessary authority to write to Professor Halford of the Melbourne University for a copy of his treatise on the subject of SNAKE BITES, and to request him to send the appliances he recommends for the purpose of carrying out his mode of treatment, which cannot be procured in this colony.

Brisbane Brothels

Of all the health legislation passed by the Queensland parliament, the measure that created the greatest controversy was the Act for the Prevention of Contagious Diseases of 1868. Its purpose was to reduce the incidence of venereal disease by compulsory medical examination of prostitutes. Some women who were found suffering from these diseases could be detained in hospital for up to six months, or more if necessary. Penalties for offences against the act included imprisonment. The legislation was based on English laws introduced to lessen the effects of venereal disease on members of the army and navy.

In England, the legislation was proclaimed only in certain areas where there were concentrations of members of the armed forces. The legislation was initiated in Queensland after Governor Bowen had been approached by British army authorities in Melbourne. Opinion on the legislation became polarized with both sides feeling very strongly about it. Many groups wanted its immediate repeal; others held staunchly for its retention. The battle raged for over half a century. In 1879, Dr Hobbs, a medical officer appointed under the act, claimed in a report to parliament that the legislation had curbed the disease. But the antagonists were not satisfied. In 1884, there began a vigorous campaign for abolition of the legislation. It consisted of letters to the press, the formation of the Social Purity Society under the chairmanship of Bishop Hale, and the forwarding of several petitions to parliament for the repeal of the act. One petition came from 3,521 women of Queensland and said the act was unjust, degrading, demoralizing, cruel, and a failure. The *Brisbane Courier* was forthright in its support for the act, while an opposition paper, *Queensland Figaro*, was just as adamant about its repeal. Attempts in 1884 in the Legislative Assembly and again in 1886 to have the act repealed resulted in an even vote each time with the Speaker giving a casting vote with the repealers. But no action was taken to put these votes into effect. In the community, the abolitionists continued their campaign but it was not until 1911 that they won their battle. Two commissioners of health, Ham in 1907, and Elkington in 1911, said the act was not having the desired medical effect. The proclamation of the act in Brisbane was rescinded on 24 August 1911. It was replaced by less controversial provisions when the Health Act was amended in the same year.

The letters quoted below set out the thoughts of some in the community when the bill was first before parliament. They were published in the *Brisbane Courier,* the first two in October 1867, and the latter two in January 1868.

AM I MY SISTER'S KEEPER?

To the Editor of the Brisbane Courier

Sir, — The reply to the above question must be in the negative by those legislators who wish the so-called "Prevention of Contagious Bill" to become law. Such a bill is a humiliating sight to see light at all, and to make it law will be a national disgrace.

If such a bill is required why not call it by its right name viz, "A Bill for the Encouragement of Dissipation, and for the Protection of Debauchery." That a contagious disease is prevalent we will not question; medical men have said so — they know, and we believe them. Tis well that suffering intimates where disease exists, otherwise we might be dead before we were aware that our end was near. So in the body social, how should we know our rottenness if there were no visible symptoms?

It is no doubt very unpleasant for young gents in their teens to suffer from this lewd leprosy. It is very inconvenient for the faithless rake, who just gets home to his uxorious wife before daylight, to find such unpleasant consequences after his dissipation. It is very disagreeable for the old hoary lecher whose hairs are grey, but whose vices luxuriate in rank greenness, to suffer from a self-inflicted disease but, notwithstanding, it is the law of righteous retribution, that as they sow so they shall reap, while society is thus made aware of the moral putrefaction that festers in our midst.

Let the above become law so that the accommodation shall be kept clean for the patrons of the brothels, then they can violate every moral and social law with safety while they wallow like swine in animal indulgencies and gratify their craving for the seduction of more innocent creatures of the weaker sex.

Has it come to this, sir, that the influence and purity of our holy religion is so far gone, and so weak in a christian land, that it is utterly powerless in compelling its professors to put on a decent garb and avoid the greatest sins. Do our moralists acknowledge that public opinion is unfit to cope with this evil and is neither so pure, so high, so fixed as to be able to restrain self indulgence, and that everyone, however depraved and vitiated, may do that which is right in his own eyes. If so, this bill weakens the public virtue still more by ignoring the moral pollution, and throwing the shield of law over the debaucher, protecting him from physical pollution in his profligacy. Let the abominable thing be thrown out, and its framers better taught. But if the time has come owing to the above weakness that the legislators must interfere, let the legislation be impartial in this matter, let what's sauce for the goose be sauce for the gander. Let seduction be made a felony to begin with, and let the gaol or a penal settlement be the punishment inflicted. Let the law of libel be so amended that every notorious offender, be he high or low, can be duly exposed to public detestation, for the present libel law is used and can be used to shelter vice from that scorn and reprobation it really merits. Let every house of bad fame be open to police inspection any hour of the day or night, and let the detective be authorised to bring with him at any visit an alderman of the city, a magistrate of the territory, or a minister of religion.

This would soon effect a reformation among men, a reformation among women would follow, and the reciprocal temptations which each address to the other would in some measure be withdrawn.

But above all, let the virtuous women of the city give to the men who are known to be guilty in this matter the cold shoulder, and show they detest both the crime and the criminal.

A CITIZEN

CONTAGIOUS DISEASES PREVENTION BILL

To the Editor of the Brisbane Courier

Sir, — Your correspondent, "Citizen", upon this subject, has thrown off, I think at random, his views.

Whether he be aware of it or not, disease is awfully prevalent in Brisbane; disease of the worst type, most difficult to cure — I will go so far as to say of an incurable character, not confined to the guilty parties; were it so, I would not have moved in the matter, not even to write a letter, but when it is known that this peculiar disease is transmitted by parents to their offspring and that the virus thus transmitted acts in the constitution of the offspring as it does — that law is most religious that prevents physical suffering by civil enactments.

Disease of this sort, when brought into the lodging-house or the home, will, under a variety of ways, inoculate others. Infection may take place when the clothes are passing through the wash tub, and persons perfectly innocent may be made bitterly to suffer for the evil-doings of others. I look upon the bill now before the House upon this subject as one of the most valuable ever introduced into the House. "Citizen" thinks the fear of consequences being removed, there will be greater indulgencies in the evil. I think the reverse; the taint of this disease from the passions, and lust burns alike in those who have indulged in illicit intercourse, and even in their offspring — something

akin to drunkenness and the effects experienced by the offspring of drunkards — for this there is no remedy that I know of equal to prevention. "Citizen" reads a chapter on morality and religion, and would have us conclude with him that the disease which sometimes the guilty contract will inspire such a wholesome dread of itself as to deter men from indulging in the sin. To this I reply, "The worm that never dies, and the fire that never shall be quenched" are awful realities, yet the fear of enduring such torments does not operate to keep men from sinning; nor is the virtue worthy the name that is to be distinguished by the fear of consequences.
Yours, &c

A VILE NUISANCE

To the Editor of the Brisbane Courier

Sir, — The prevalence of prostitution is a fact which is likely to perplex our social reformers for some time to come. Perhaps we in Brisbane have not more reason to complain that have other metropolitan cities. It is a source of disease, of physical and moral wretchedness, which it is apparently hopeless to think of quite closing, and difficult for legislation appreciably to diminish. Admitting this is however, a very different thing from what there appears to be in modern times a tendency to do — that is, to make the impossibility of altogether suppressing it become a kind of justification of it, so that one of the cardinal sins may have a prospect of reaching the status of "an institution".

Last week I was amazed to discover that in a line with our business premises in Elizabeth Street, and only separated from them by sixty-six feet of fencing, a low brothel had commenced operation. Exactly opposite this was another, where ginger-beer was ostensibly sold. All passengers could see at once what these places really were. Behind the ginger-beer shop, are four cottages belonging to a man named, I believed Byrne, who, I am told, is at the diggings. These four cottages front the building formerly known as the Leader office, and from the door of our stores is plainly visible all that goes on outside these cottages, and a good deal of what goes on inside, as the doors are always open. The wife and family of the landlord live in one of these cottages; the other three are, I believe, brothels. They are conveniently accessible from both Queen Street and from Elizabeth Street; from Queen Street by the corner of Messrs Dickson and Duncan's auction mart; at this corner the wretched inmates solicit at night. One of them was seen last Thursday morning to pass from the front door of one of the cottages to the privy directly opposite, with nothing on her person but a chemise; and, indeed, this appears to be the only garment considered necessary to wear until they dress at night to ply their filthy occupation.

I have written to the Police Magistrate and spoken to the police and am pleased in being able to say that they have expressed a hearty wish to do all that is in their power to extinguish this intolerable and — to us commercially — highly injurious nuisance. But, they inform me — what many besides me will probably be surprised to learn — that the means of remedy in their hands are miserably inefficient. It appears that the Queensland Towns Police Act is by no means the vigorous capable measure the Victoria Act for similar purposes is. In Melbourne the police have power to maintain a vigilant domiciliary surveillance over brothels and disreputable houses; and any failure or neglect in its exercise is regarded by the Judges of Victoria as a serious breach of police duty.

The Police Magistrate and the police of Brisbane complain in strong terms of their hands being tied in this matter of requisite jurisdiction over brothels. They assure me that they can do next to nothing to conserve public decency; unless they travel beyond and exceed the law as it at present stands. This is greatly discreditable to the citizens of Brisbane and to the colony generally and calls loudly for amendment. I have seen a bill to amend the Towns Police Act in these respects, and informed that it would, with perhaps some modifications, have probably been passed through Parliament but for the last change of Ministry. May I be permitted to suggest to some members of the Legislative Assembly the advisability of promptly bringing this bill forward, or one to the same effect, before the present Session closes. It is not necessary to add an expression of my feeling, that the necessity of writing such a letter as this ought not to have existed, and my earnest hope that it may be at once destroyed.

WILLIAM BROOKES
Brisbane, January 11

THE SOCIAL EVIL
To the Editor of the Brisbane Courier

Sir, — In reference to the above heading and the very able letter of Mr. William Brookes on the subject, I desire to say a few words. Within the last few months a brothel of the lowest order has sprung into existence a few yards from my residence, the annoyance of which I leave you to picture to yourself — suffice for me to say that the screeching and yelling issuing from the same are anything but desirable; but this is not the worst part of the nuisance complained of; — my house has more than once, at midnight, been taken for a place of the kind.

I have spoken to the police on the subject, who, I am pleased to say, have shown every desire to put down the nuisance, but at the same time expressed their inability to do so.

This sort thing should not be allowed to exist to the annoyance of the community, and, in conclusion, I have only to express a hope that our law makers will take such steps as will suppress the evil so very generally complained of.

Enclosed I beg to hand you my card.

VERITAS
Brisbane, January 13

From Convict to Doctor

"Put forward Kevin Izod O'Doherty" was the order given on 3 November 1848 in the Commission Court, Green Street, Dublin. As Mr Justice Crampton, the presiding judge, waited for it to be obeyed, a well-built, good-looking young Irishman entered the raised dock. The judge began his pre-sentence speech:

> Kevin Izod O'Doherty, you were indicted for compassing the deposition of Her Majesty, the Queen, and also for compassing to levy war against Her Majesty, in order by force and constraint to compel her to change her measures and counsels. You have been acquitted on all the counts charging the former intent, and have been found guilty of compassing to levy war against Her Majesty, the Queen, for the purpose of compelling her by force and constraint to change her measures and counsels.

Judge Crampton concluded his harangue:

> I fear I must add, that I cannot conceive, I have never read any publications more dangerous, more wicked, more clearly designed to excite insurrection, rebellion and revolution than those publications which have emanated from your press, and of which you have been ascertained, by the verdict of your jury to be the guilty publisher. Under these circumstances, the Court feels called on to pronounce upon you the sentence, that you be transported for ten years.

Quite unperturbed by the sentence just passed, O'Doherty requested and was granted permission to speak. He pointed out that "he was influenced but by one feeling, and had but one object in view. He felt deeply for the sufferings and privations endured by his fellow-countrymen and desired by every means consistent with a manly and honourable resistance to put an end to those sufferings". He concluded by saying that "out of twelve jurors permitted to be sworn there was not one Roman Catholic".

As O'Doherty was led away to the vaulted passage connecting the court with Newgate Prison, a beautiful, raven-haired Irish colleen rushed to his side and whispered, "Have faith. I'll wait." She was Mary Eva Kelly, known as "Eva of the Nation".

Kevin O'Doherty was born, the son of a Dublin solicitor, on 7 September 1823 and commenced the study of medicine in 1842.

Records show that he was a diligent student and in 1848 on completion of his training, the famous physician William Stokes certified that "O'Doherty was qualified to undertake the charge of a medical institution". However, in addition to walking the wards of the famous Meath Hospital where he undertook his clinical instruction, he had time to take an active interest in the affairs of the Young Ireland Movement. This movement had grown up around the editors of a newspaper called the *Nation*. They were Charles Duffy, Thomas Davis and John Dillon.

The greatest political figure in Ireland of the time was Daniel O'Connell, who was given the name of "The Great Liberator" for the part he played in winning emancipation for the Irish Catholics. O'Connell then commenced a campaign to have the Union of England and Ireland repealed. The Young Irelanders at first threw their weight behind O'Connell, but then left to form a separate organization — The Irish Confederation — when he declined to use force to achieve his objective. For several months the confederation held meetings and published newspapers which condemned the British and urged the Irish to overthrow the foreign yoke. But in 1848, the Young Irelanders planned active rebellion. O'Doherty's main contribution was to publish the *Irish Tribune* with a fellow medical student, Dalton Williams. The first issue appeared a few weeks before O'Doherty was due to sit for his final examinations in medicine. The following quotations amply demonstrate the purpose of the paper.

> Shall we, with folded arms, witness our jackal foe drive from our fields our sheep and our oxen and the corn thereof to thrive and fatten upon?
>
> Forbid it Heaven. No; the strong men of this land, by the concentrated fire of revenge, are uged to save the coming harvest and ease their longing thirst deep, deep in the blood of the English foe.
>
> We call on the people of Dublin, as they value their lives, their liberties and the happiness of their homes . . . to take this matter into their hands . . . to tell this Royal Lady . . . that the Crown, which will stand in the way of righting and ruling themselves . . . must perish.

The inevitable clash with the British came. The Habeas Corpus Act was suspended and many of the Young Ireland leaders were arrested. O'Doherty was caught in this drive and instead of graduating in medicine found himself in Newgate Prison.

In prison, the Young Irelanders were visited by female supporters. One of these was Eva Kelly, a native of Galway who had come to Dublin to be near the centre of the attempt to expel the English. Eva Kelly was proud of her rebel ancestry. She was descendant of the great O'Kelly sept of Ui Maine, who were one of the dangerous Irish septs named by the local authority, the Corporation of Galway. The corporation, in 1518, issued an order that "Neither O nor Mac shall strut or swagger through the streets of Galway". A more specific instruction was promulgated forbidding the citizens of the town to admit into their houses Burkes, MacWilliams, Kellys or any other sept. On Eva's mother's side there was rebel stock also, for she was an O'Flaherty. Over the Galway city gates was once inscribed, "God deliver us from the fury of the O'Flahertys". In her early teens Eva Kelly demonstrated that she had considerable literary talent and was composing poems of a high standard. Having the ancestry described above, and an uncle who had sympathy for the Young Ireland cause, it is not surprising that she was soon contributing nationalistic poems to the *Nation*. The regular appearance of poems under the pseudonym of "Eva" soon won her the

Former Irish rebel Kevin O'Doherty came to Queensland in 1862 and practised medicine in Ipswich and Brisbane. (Courtesy Oxley Library)

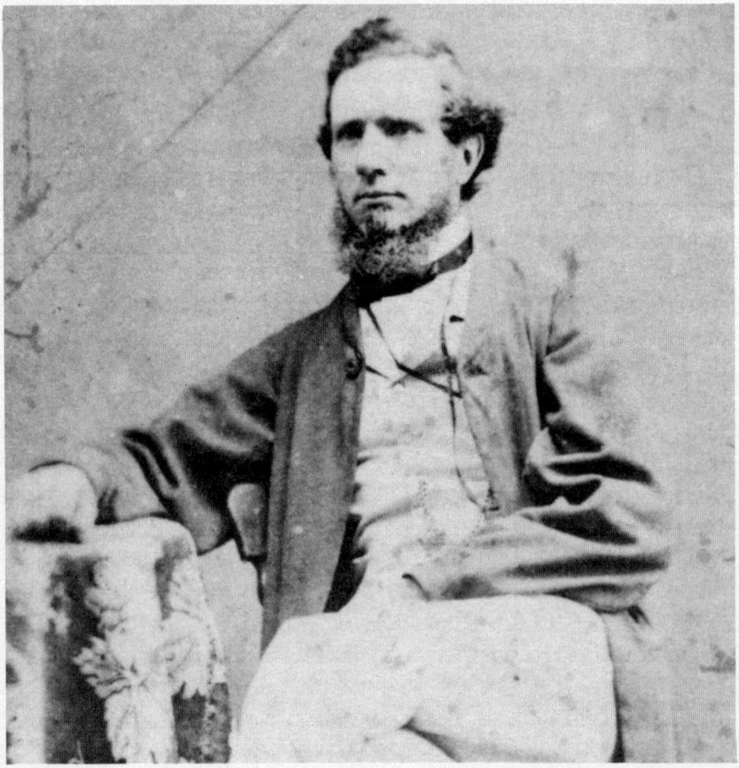

title "Eva of The Nation". A typical verse from her poem, "Down Britannia" reads:

> Down, Britannia, brigand down
> No more to rule with sceptred hand.
> Truth raises o'er thy throne and crown
> Her exorcising wand
> I see the "writing on the wall".
> The proud, the thrice-accursed shall fall.
> Down, Britannia, down.

P.J. Smyth, one of the Young Irelanders, makes the following reference in his memoirs to the development of the romance between Eva and Kevin O'Doherty whilst Kevin was an inmate of Newgate Prison.

> Like many members of the party Kevin had been visited by Miss Bruton. On one occasion she took with her a young girl, Miss Kelly, who at the time was charming everyone by the sweetness of her poems. Tall, with dark, dreamy eyes and wonderful black hair, reaching to her knees, poor O'Doherty fell a victim to her charms. One visit followed another and became a weekly occurrence. . . Their farewell was a touching one, Eva promising to remain faithful and with a hope that he might come back to claim the promise she now gave him to be his wife.

O'Doherty was tried three times. The first two juries disagreed and were dismissed. O'Doherty was then approached by the British authorities with a promise of freedom provided he would set an example of debasing himself. If he would plead guilty he would not be called for judgment. For himself there was only one answer to be given to this insulting offer — to treat it with disdain. But, what about Eva? If he accepted, he would be free to sit for his final medical examinations in a few weeks and then marry Eva. When he consulted her, he found he should not have had any doubt about her thoughts on the matter. Her advice to her lover was, "Be true to Ireland, and I'll be true to you". The British offer was scornfully rejected. Kevin next appeared on trial at the end of October 1848. This time the jury returned a verdict of guilty.

Not long after his conviction O'Doherty was transferred to Richmond Prison, further from the centre of Dublin. Here, too, were imprisoned other leaders: Smith O'Brien, Meagher, McManus, Martin and O'Donohue. Earlier, another Young Irelander, Mitchel, had been transported to Bermuda. The prisoners were kept at Richmond another six months. Then, early one morning in the middle of June 1849, O'Doherty and Martin were taken from the prison in a van guarded by a body of mounted police and a regiment of dragoons with loaded carbines and swords drawn. The convoy set off at a gallop along the deserted streets of Dublin to Kingstown. There the prisoners were placed on board the war steamer, *Trident* to take them to Spike Island in Cork Harbour. At Cork, they were transferred to the *Mount Stewart Elphinstone* carrying 230 convicts to Moreton Bay. The *Mount Stewart Elphinstone* was a far better ship than many of the previous convict transports and special quarters had been installed for the state prisoners. Four months after leaving Cork, the vessel arrived in Sydney Harbour where O'Doherty and Martin were transferred to the brig *Emma* bound for the notorious convict island, Van Diemen's Land. The two prisoners were apprehensive about their future on arrival there. Would they be treated as common convicts and sent to Port Arthur, the most feared of all the convict settlements from where warning of attempted escape was given by dogs held at intervals across Eaglehawk Neck?

Their lot, however was far better than they had expected. On arrival, O'Doherty and Martin and five other Irish rebels who came in other ships, were offered ticket-of-leave conditions on the understanding that they would not take advantage of the comparative liberty to escape. All except Smith O'Brien accepted the offer. Smith O'Brien was incarcerated first on Maria Island and later at Port Arthur, where his cottage is included in the tourist attractions today. The exiles were expected to observe the following regulations: they were confined to the district allocated; they had to report regularly to the police magistrate; observe a curfew of 10 p.m. and not frequent theatres or billiard rooms.

Back in Ireland, Eva suffered months of despair. She couldn't lift a pen as she feared for Kevin's safety. This unhappy mood was only lightened by news from Kevin that he had not been shipwrecked or treated as a common convict as she was sure would be the case, but was living with a Tipperary man, John Ryan, at Oatlands about fifty miles north of Hobart. When she did pick up the pen again she wrote of her love and their separation:

THE PATH ACROSS THE SEA
My love, my hope, my longing
Make a path across the sea,
I can reach thee. I can clasp there
Although parted we may be.

Naught can come between us, dearest —
Naught can hold thee back from me!

The holder of a ticket-of-leave was expected to support himself in the community to which he had been allocated. Kevin was unable to find suitable employment in Oatlands. In desperation, he applied to have his ticket-of-leave revoked so he could exist at one of the convict settlements. He was persuaded not to do so by his friends. Soon after, he was allowed to transfer to Hobart where he worked with Dr Crooke and then for two years was an assistant surgeon at St Mary's Hospital. While there, he was apprehended for being outside the bounds of his district during a visit to Smith O'Brien, then living at New Norfolk, after accepting ticket-of-leave. As a result, O'Doherty spent three weeks as a common convict splitting roof shingles in a chain-gang. In the middle of 1854, news came of a conditional pardon for Smith O'Brien, Martin and O'Doherty. The four other Irish exiles had escaped to America. The condition in the pardon prohibited the exiles from returning to England, Scotland or Ireland. The three rebels, accompanied by P.J. Smyth, who had gone to Van Diemen's Land to engineer an escape for Smith O'Brien, left immediately for Melbourne where they were feted by Irish-born citizens. O'Doherty and Smyth decided to try their luck on the Victorian goldfields. After no success, O'Doherty made secret arrangements to travel incognito on the *James Baines,* a gold clipper bound to sail for Liverpool around Cape Horn.

When he arrived in England, a fellow passenger reported O'Doherty's illegal presence in England. However, he managed to escape detection, and travelled to Galway in Ireland where he and Eva spent a few joyful days in a wonderful reunion. The sub-inspector of police at Galway advised Dublin Castle that "it was whispered abroad that a strange gentleman was staying with the Kelly family". But again Kevin was able to slip away without any action being taken against him. The couple were secretly married in London in August 1855 and went to Paris. Here O'Doherty worked at the Pitie Hospital and studied at the Paris Anatomy School. Then, to their great joy, in 1856 a full pardon was granted. The couple returned to Dublin immediately and Kevin began to prepare for his final examinations in medicine. In 1857, nine years later than first anticipated, Kevin graduated from the College of Surgeons, Ireland.

In the course of a busy practice that followed, O'Doherty made firm friends with Rev. Dr James Quinn. Although he was quite successful in practice, Kevin always had thoughts of emigrating to Australia. When Quinn was appointed Bishop of Brisbane, the young couple made definite plans. After arriving in Australia at the end of 1860, O'Doherty practised in Sydney until Quinn took up his appointment in Brisbane. He came to Queensland and was registered as a medical practitioner in the young colony on 3 March 1862. For three years he practised in Ipswich. Shortly after his arrival he demonstrated a loyalty to Bishop Quinn which he maintained for twenty years. He strongly supported the bishop in a dispute with Father McGinty, the parish priest, over church funds. Moving to Brisbane in 1865, O'Doherty set up practice in George Street. For two decades, he was to be prominent in many fields — medical, political, church and public affairs.

There is ample evidence to show that O'Doherty was a very sound doctor. In 1866, he was appointed an honorary visiting surgeon to the Brisbane Hospital when it was still situated in George Street on the site of the present Supreme Court. He held this position for several years after the hospital was built the next year at Bowen Bridge Road. He pioneered operations at a time when surgery was just developing and one reads of operations being delayed until the respected surgeon arrived. He was always willing to travel into the bush to see patients, going on one occasion on horseback to the Tweed River to attend a timbergetter seriously injured by a falling tree. The medical profession indicated its esteem by electing him president of the Queensland Medical Society in 1882. The government appointed him a member of the Medical Board of Queensland and the Central Board of Health.

In 1867, he was elected one of the three members representing north Brisbane in the Legislative Assembly. The number of electors was not large, and counting was complete an hour or so after voting closed. On election day, O'Doherty was called out of town on a professional visit just as the counting commenced. He often told the story of how, on returning to the town, he asked a passer-by how the voting went. Back came the answer in a North of Ireland brogue, "Bad enough, that bloody papist, O'Doherty, got in." He threw in his lot with the "Town Liberals" and once told the electors that they should "rejoice in the prospect of escape from the positive evil of the squatting rule".

O'Doherty was to the forefront when debates on health matters were being held. He introduced the first Health Act to be passed by the Queensland parliament, and was either a member of or gave expert evidence before select committees on health subjects. He was interested in many subjects and in the debate on education he reflected Bishop Quinn's desire to have state aid for denominational schools continued. When the battle was lost, O'Doherty, in protest, declined to serve on the government's education board to which he had been appointed. He resigned his seat in the lower house in 1873 due to the pressure of his professional practice but was elected a member of the Legislative Council in 1877. Soon after, he was involved in a bitter debate with Dr William Hobbs, another member of the upper house, over a report of a royal commission on the Woogaroo Lunatic Asylum and Reception Houses. No doubt the rest of the house enjoyed the dispute between the two medical members. In 1881, the Irish doctor courageously introduced a pharmacy bill to give chemists their own board despite strenuous opposition by his colleagues on the medical board and the profession generally.

Bishop Quinn's autocratic manner brought many enemies among his priests, the laity and the community. However, O'Doherty was prepared to speak in the bishop's favour no matter what the occasion. At a function in 1869 when the first Brisbane Grammar School, built in Roma Street, was opened by Governor Blackall, O'Doherty, a trustee of the school, startled the audience by remarking on the absence of the Catholic and Anglican bishops, who had not been invited. He said that he himself would not have come if he had known the bishops were not to be asked. Despite an anti-Quinn faction, the Irish doctor remained the leading Catholic layman for twenty years. He was in the official party when the new St Stephen's Cathedral was consecrated in 1874. He had strongly supported its building and gave generously to the funds for its erection.

O'Doherty often remarked on the tolerance among colonists to one another, no matter what their origin was. However, when testing time came, he demonstrated that strong Irish nationalism which was first seen in his student days and which never left him. It was O'Doherty, who, in 1875, suggested that a centenary celebration in honour of Daniel O'Connell be held in Brisbane. At an enthusiastic function it was O'Doherty who delivered the oration in memory of the Great Liberator. When the news of the 1879 famine in Ireland reached Queensland, O'Doherty chaired the first meeting to organize a relief fund. Working with John Flood, a Fenian rebel transported to Western Australia in 1867, but then in Queensland under a conditional pardon, O'Doherty initiated a campaign which raised £12,000 to send to his native land to help his starving countrymen. During these years, the colony's newspapers always prominently featured news from the British Isles. A new leader in Ireland, Parnell, was campaigning for Home Rule for his country. The *Brisbane Courier* adopted a strong anti-Parnell attitude. Despite this, and while some prominent Irishmen held back, O'Doherty showed his mettle. He chaired not only the Queensland branch of the Irish National League but when the Irish members of parliament, the Redmond brothers, visited to raise funds for Home Rule, he presided over a national convention in Melbourne.

During her life in Australia, Eva was less prominent than she had been in Ireland. Of course, the stimulus to write nationalistic poems as she had done in early life in Ireland was no longer present. She was a busy housewife with a husband and family to care for. However, her pen was not completely idle. When she did compose new verse, the subjects indicated her adopted country as is seen in her poem, "Queensland".

Thou art in sooth a lovely land
As fair as ever fancy painted,
In virgin freshness calm and bland
By shadows dark untainted.
But Ah! Upon that bright expanse
The glory of a dim Elysian,
'Tis but a cold and soulless glance
That meets the gazer's vision.

Of eight children born to the couple only five survived to adulthood — four sons and one daughter. Of the four boys, the eldest, William, qualified as a dentist in America and worked for a while with his uncle in Dublin. He returned to Australia with his brother Edward, who had just graduated from the Irish College of Surgeons. The third boy, Vincent, was a bank officer and the fourth son, Kevin, managed his father's sugar plantation on the Johnstone River in North Queensland. In 1882, Dr O'Doherty built a fourteen-room house in Ann Street which he called Frascati after the area in which his mother had lived in Dublin in her later years. There were three consulting rooms on the ground floor, two occupied by himself and son Edward in their medical partnership, with William, the dentist, using the third. The house later became the nurses home for St Martin's Hospital.

Kevin's efforts on behalf of the Home Rule cause and his participation in Queensland politics attracted Parnell's attention and, in 1885, he was invited to Ireland with the idea of becoming a member of the Irish National Party at the next election. He saw an opportunity to help once again in the cause which had failed in

1848 and he readily accepted the invitation. On his arrival in his native land he was treated as a hero. On 1 September 1885, the Freedom of the City of Dublin was bestowed on him. At the Meath convention on 8 October he was selected as a candidate for North Meath, which he later won at the general election. This was followed by an invitation to give a public lecture at the Rotunda. During a brief visit to Australia to put his affairs in order before he took his seat in the House of Commons, he was guest of honour at numerous banquets and functions in Brisbane, Sydney and Melbourne. In Brisbane, however, the banquet was boycotted by most of the establishment, much to the delight of the *Brisbane Courier*. Returning to Ireland, he took his place in the Commons with the Parnell Party. His maiden speech in the

Dr Kevin O'Doherty, president of the Queensland Medical Society, in 1882. (Courtesy AMA [Queensland Branch])

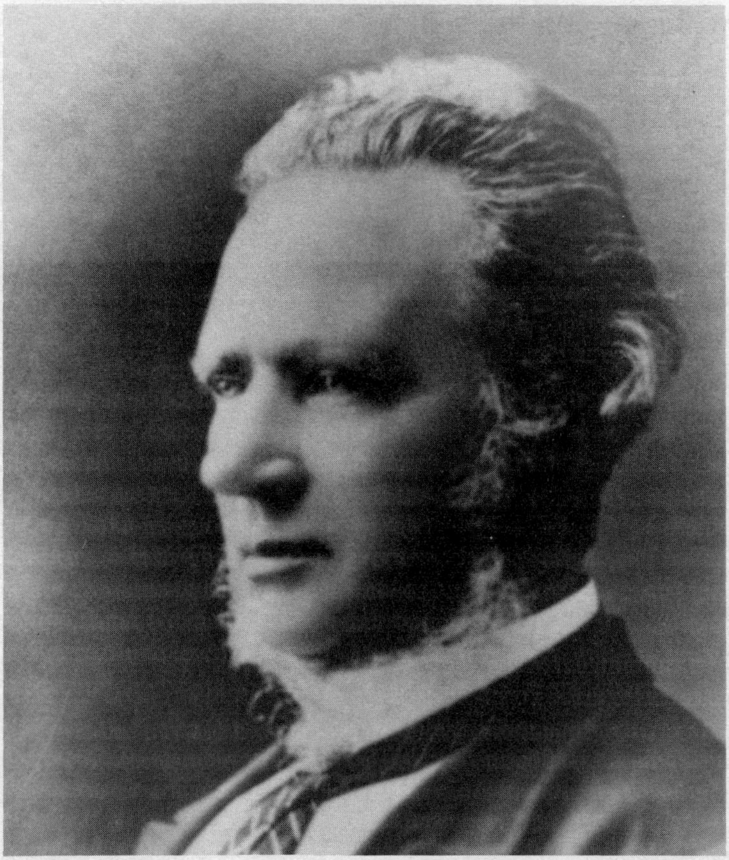

Home Rule debate was received with much acclaim by his Irish colleagues. He was riding the crest of a wave.

But, his triumph was shortlived. When the vote was taken on 8 June 1886, the Home Rule bill was lost and Gladstone resigned. This marked a turning point in O'Doherty's career. From then on, there was great sadness in the lives of Kevin and Eva. He declined to be renominated in the ensuing election. In his letter of resignation from the party, he stated that "only imperative private reasons" prevented him from accepting. It is most likely that the "imperative private reasons" were financial difficulties. Returning quietly to Brisbane which he had left in a blaze of glory, he soon went to Sydney where for a while he was a member of the honorary staff of St Vincent's Hospital. Then, in 1887, at the age of sixty-four, he was appointed government medical officer at Croydon in North Queensland, where gold had been recently discovered. It is suggested he chose the position to try to balance his account by a lucky strike. In this he was unsuccessful and he returned to Brisbane in 1890 with the coffers empty.

For the next fifteen years until O'Doherty's death in 1905, the fates were very cruel to the Irish doctor and his wife. He made an attempt to enter private practice again, but, this too failed. The Queensland government, remembering how well he had served the community in the past, alleviated the couple's plight by appointing Kevin to part-time positions. In a few years blindness prevented him carrying out his duties. Three colleagues, John Thomson, Espie Dods and John Flynn, who held the ageing doctor in high esteem, performed his work while he received the salary. The estimates for the home department list him in these positions until he was seventy-seven. The fine home in Ann Street had to be sold and the couple retired to Bayswater Street in Rosalie. But, other sadness was heaped on them. Their sons, so full of promise, died one by one in the last decade of the nineteenth century. At last, on 15 July 1905, the great man breathed his last, his address then being Heussler Terrace, Milton. Typical of the many tributes paid to him in obituary notices is the following from the *Brisbane Age*:

> There was nothing that was not large, generous and open-minded in the character of the well-known doctor. In truth, it was this wholesome freedom from hypocritical restraint which caused him the troubles of his life.

Eva lived for another five years in straitened circumstances. Her only surviving child, Gertrude, and her only grandson lived with her. Her letters to Father Hickey in Yorkshire tell of her loneliness and great sadness at being neglected by the Irish for whom she and her husband had attempted so much. It was during this period, at the age of seventy-six, she wrote the poem which depicts the great sorrow that was hers when one after another she lost first her four sons and finally her beloved husband.

TENEBRAE

Night's solemn hour! Upon the holy fane,
The mystic lights upon the altar burn,
And voices chanting in a sad refrain,
Unceasing seem to mourn —
When lo! with sudden smite,
Is quenched one shining light.
One light has vanished from the holy fane.

Thus one by one in gathering fear and gloom
The phantom voices murmuring low between,
Each light goes out with fatal stroke of doom
Until upon the scene
A dismal darkness falls,
A silence that appals,
The darkness and the silence of the tomb!

In 1910, Eva died at the age of eighty years. The only grandson was killed in France during World War I, fighting with the Australian forces. There was no male to carry on this line of the O'Doherty name. Gertrude, the only child to survive her famous parents, married Inspector O'Sullivan of the Queensland Police Force. They had no children. Colleen Melhuish, a descendent of O'Sullivan's first marriage, provided valuable material for the preparation of this history. Mignon O'Doherty, a granddaughter of Kevin and Eva, went to London and achieved success as an actress in the original cast of Agatha Christie's play *The Mousetrap*, and other plays. Prudence Chapman, a daughter of Mignon's, lives in London, and two granddaughters, Caroline and Vivienne Nesbitt, live in New Hampshire in the United States of America.

And so the Irish medico and his poet wife were laid to rest. Theirs was no ordinary life. They survived many hardships: Kevin's transportation with its heartbreaking separation; the nine years' delay in his graduation as a doctor; emigration to a new land; the loss of their children; the financial difficulties; and finally Kevin's blindness. But they were made of stern stuff.

They lived for eighty years despite all these vicissitudes and enjoyed many triumphs. Their lives were lived on a higher plane than most and they lifted to that plane many who lived around them. Tom MacBride, the Caloundra poet, epitomized their lives in a sonnet he wrote after their story was told him. He entitled it *So Much for Love*.

SO MUCH FOR LOVE

So much for love! Two spirits rare, conjoin'd —
  Emancipators, Aye, — Glory foregone!
Life's sweets by sullen grief so oft purloin'd!
  Far distant tracks, and strange to journey on!
Exponent was he of the healer's art
  Of tremendous use to his fellow man
In other spheres he played an equal part
  Suchwise as only true philosophers can.
And she, the sparkling light of his life
  To record it so by the power of the muse.
Was ever man bless'd with a dearer wife
  Than would sing his praise as the Gods would choose?
Bricks both, glazed in the fires of tribulation —
  Bright keystones in the building of our nation.

Admirers of O'Doherty and his wife erected a monument to their memory in the Toowong cemetery. The inscription reads:

Sacred
To the memory of
KEVIN IZOD O'DOHERTY
The Irish patriot
Died 15 July 1905, aged 81 years
Whose name will live in Irish History
And whose memory ever remains enshrined
In Irish hearts at Home and Abroad
Also his gifted wife
EVA OF THE NATION

Physician and Muse, man and wife!
They came from Ireland's shores.
Through adversity their light shone brightly,
Inspiring all on whom it shone.
Their like never die but live into eternity.

Tinkering in the Bush

In the days when the only means of travel to parts of Queensland was by horse or bullock dray, people living in communities too small to support a medical practitioner often experienced great difficulty obtaining medical aid. At times, their needs were satisfied to a degree by men whose names did not appear on the Queensland medical board register. Some of these held foreign diplomas not recognized in Queensland, while others followed various occupations but used medical skills picked up in all sorts of ways to help in emergencies. While the communities were grateful for such help and sometimes even government officers used the services of such men, the registered practitioners generally frowned on such activities. One member of the medical establishment who felt strongly about the matter was Kevin O'Doherty, a leading Brisbane medico and a member of parliament representing North Brisbane. O'Doherty's attitude is illustrated in the following story from the pages of Hansard.

In the Legislative Assembly on 19 December 1871, O'Doherty, who was one of the representatives for North Brisbane said that:

> He rose for the purpose of moving the adjournment of the House, with the view of bringing under the attention of the House, and of the honorable members of the Government, a statement which appeared in the "Brisbane Courier" of the previous day — a statement which consisted of a portion of the evidence of Sergeant Downie, at the magisterial investigation held at St. George, with relation to the murder of Mr Zieman. In the report of the investigation in yesterday's "Courier", he found the following statement as part of the evidence of Sergeant Downie:—
>
> "I left Constable Henry in charge of the body; on the morning of the 29th, I assisted Dr Godfrey to make a further examination of the body; we stripped the whole of the clothes off on that occasion; the trousers and braces produced are those I took off the body; in my presence, Dr Godfrey removed the head from the body, and an hour afterwards the neck; I afterwards escorted the head and neck into Surat; the remaining portion of the body was then buried about 200 yards from where it was found".
>
> He had no means of ascertaining the exact amount of truth that was contained in the statement; but as it consisted of the sworn testimony

of a sergeant of police, he thought it was his duty to call the attention of the Government to the matter; and he thought it was highly important that the attention of the Government should be directed to it. There were two circumstances connected with the case which he could not but regard as monstrous. The one was, that the body should have been so abominably mutilated as the body of Mr Zieman seemed to have been; and the other was, that Mr Godfrey was not a legally qualified practitioner. He (Dr O'Doherty) had taken the trouble to make enquiries at the Medical Board as to Mr Godfrey, and he found that there was not a medical man of that name on the list of legally qualified practitioners. Now, this man, was nevertheless, allowed, in the presence of Government officials, to cut off the head, in the first instance, and then to cut off the neck, of Mr Zieman. The head and neck were placed in a tin box, and taken into Surat, and the other portion of the body was buried two hundred yards from where it was found. . . He did not see that there was any necessity whatever in the interests of justice that there should have been such a mutilation of the body of Mr Zieman. . . He could inform the House, that any properly qualified medical man could at once, on examination, have certified as to the cause of death, without mutilating the body in the way that Mr Zieman's body had been mutilated. Why, he would ask, should any tinker that might be found in the bush be allowed to mutilate the body of a human being a such a way; and why should the life of a fellow being be left dependent upon such evidence? But this was not the first case of the kind that had occurred recently. Within the last twelve months a case of a similar nature took place — similar to this extent, that a man who was not a legally qualified medical practitioner was called upon to give evidence on a critical case in which the accuracy of the medical testimony involved the liberty of a fellow-citizen. Now he held that it was quite contrary to the spirit of all justice, that the evidence of any tinker who might be picked up in the bush should be received as to the cause of death, seeing that upon his evidence might depend the life of a fellow-man. He had only to say further, in conclusion, that he thought it was the duty of the Government to institute inquiries as to why the body of Mr Zieman was so mutilated, and why Mr Godfrey was called upon to make examination as to the cause of death.

The Premier and Colonial Secretary [the Hon. A.H. Palmer, later Sir Arthur] said, "If Mr Godfrey, as asserted, was not a legally qualified medical man, he could not give evidence at the trial as to the cause of death; and, therefore, it was necessary that the skull should be sent down for evidence as to the cause of death at the trial of the parties for the murder of Mr Zieman."

Mr Miles (Member for Maranoa which included Surat) said he fully agreed with the honorable member for North Brisbane, Dr O'Doherty, that there was no necessity for the mutilation of the body of Mr Zieman. He did not see that it was at all necessary for the ends of justice that the head should have been cut off, and then the neck, and that those portions of the body should have been sealed up in a tin case, and sent down under escort to Surat. He believed that evidence of Mr Buttenshaw, and of the members of the police force, who were present when the body was found, would have been quite sufficient to satisfy any jury as to the cause of death; and he held, therefore, that it was quite unnecessary that the body should have been mutilated as it had been. The honorable member for North Brisbane, Dr O'Doherty, had spoken of Mr Godfrey as a tinker. Well, he was not prepared, from his knowledge, to say what Mr Godfrey was, but he could say from good authority in Surat — and his authority was a gentleman in the public service — that Mr Godfrey was a highly qualified medical man, and a very skilful practitioner. It seemed, however, that from some misfortune he had not passed the Medical Board in this colony, and was not, therefore, a legally qualified practitioner. But, he was a highly respectable man; and he (Mr Miles) was prepared to say that, though Mr Godfrey was not a legally qualified practitioner, he was, as a medical man, far superior to most medical gentlemen in the colony who were qualified by law. In the outlying districts of the colony, where there was not sufficient population to induce a legally qualified medical man to take up his residence, people were glad to obtain the services of gentlemen who were known to be otherwise qualified. Now, he had it on very high authority, that Mr Godfrey was a most competent medical man. To have obtained the services of a legally qualified man, in this instance, it would have been necessary to have gone a hundred miles from the scene of the murder; and there was no telegraph in the district, by which means a legally qualified medical man could have been sent for at once; and Mr Zieman had been dead two days before his body was discovered. Well, it would have taken several days to get a legally qualified medical man to go up and examine the body; and by that time, at this hot season of the year, the body would have been in a very advanced state of decomposition.

Patrick Collins, station hand, was charged with the murder and appeared before Judge Lutwyche at the Toowoomba assizes in May 1872. After a short retirement, the jury found him guilty. The judge announced the following sentence: "Patrick Collins, you have been found guilty of the foul and deliberate murder of Simon Zieman and the law adjudges you to die. I implore you not to waste your time in any fruitless efforts to escape but use it in earnest prayer for the mercy of your offended God. The Sentence of the Court is that you be taken to the place from which you came and thence to the Brisbane Gaol and within the precincts of which gaol you be hanged by the neck until you be dead, on such day as the Governor, with the advice of the Executive Council, may determine and may God Almighty have mercy on your soul."

On 26 May, the day appointed by the Executive Council, Collins was executed.

There is no evidence to show whether the government took any action on O'Doherty's complaint either in general or in particular regard to Mr Godfrey. In time, as the towns in outback Queensland became more populated, many doctors commenced practice. Their availability varied over the years that followed but with the arrival of the motor car, better roads, aeroplane and such services as the Royal Flying Doctor Service, the people in remote areas had more ready access to medical attention.

Governor in Waiting

In February 1877, the Eastern and Australian Mail Steam Company's ship, the *Brisbane*, with Captain Balfour in command, sailed out of Hong Kong harbour bound for Australia. On board was Sir Arthur Kennedy, recently appointed governor of Queensland. The task of governing a colony was not new to Sir Arthur, for he had occupied a similar position in Western Australia, Vancouver Island, West African settlements and then Hong Kong. Travelling with him was his devoted daughter, Georgina, who, since the death of her mother in 1874, acted as official hostess for His Excellency. Sir Arthur's party also included his daughter's companion, Miss Banks, and his private secretary, Captain O'Callaghan. A retinue of Chinese also came to attend to the governor's domestic wants. Later, his refusal to dismiss them made Sir Arthur unpopular with the working class of the colony. The vessel's complement included first class passengers, and many Chinese travelling steerage. The *Brisbane Courier* criticized the arrangements made to bring Sir Arthur to his new post:

> The people of Australia are looked upon in England as being a trifle too democratic, as inclined to pay too little respect to high rank and exalted dignity. Yet, when we have been called upon to do so, we have not grudged the expenditure necessary to receive a prince of the blood with the ceremonies due to his rank, nor to provide the means to enable our Governor to travel as befits Her Majesty's representatives. It is reserved for the Imperial authorities to lower the state which has always been accorded the Governor of Queensland, by sending us one, as a passenger on a merchant steamer crowded with hundreds of Chinese coolies. Such procedure does not indicate much regard for the colony nor the gentleman appoint to govern us, but if the Imperial Government chooses to abolish that ceremony and etiquette with which it has hitherto surrounded its high officers we can make no objection and must we suppose be content to register the example for future imitation.

Although the steamer was due to call at Singapore and several ports along the Queensland coast she was scheduled to reach Brisbane, the colony's capital, a few days before Good Friday at the end of March. Miss Kennedy and her companion were looking forward to spending Easter in their new home, Government House, Brisbane. All went well until the steamer left Bowen, in north Queensland. The governor and his party were then shocked to learn that one of the Chinese passengers had developed smallpox. On 24 March, the sick man was put ashore on Curtis Island with several of the people with whom he had had close contact and the steamer proceeded to Brisbane. Two days later, she anchored in Moreton Bay, where passengers would be transferred to a smaller vessel to take them up the Brisbane River to the capital.

On news of her arrival, the Queensland premier, John Douglas accompanied by several senior ministers, went down the river to meet the new governor. As they drew near they saw the yellow quarantine flag flying from the *Brisbane*'s mast. Dr Challinor, the health officer, always a man who followed the letter of the law, had already placed the vessel in quarantine. An embarrassed premier spoke to the new governor over the ship's side. He explained that not only Queensland but all Australia was most anxious about the threat of the introduction of smallpox. Sir Arthur said he "quite approved of due caution being taken, though it was his own individual opinion that in this particular case, which had to be considered, there was no cause for undue alarm". A worried premier returned up the river to Brisbane and called a hasty cabinet meeting. It was decided to appoint a medical commission consisting of three leading medical practitioners, O'Doherty, Bancroft and Cannan. They were to go down to the ship the next morning with Dr Challinor to enquire into the sanitary condition of the steamer and her passengers and advise the government regarding the safety or otherwise of releasing them from quarantine. The *Brisbane Courier* made the following scathing comments on the action being taken.

> We believe that it has been arranged that the "Kate" shall go down to the bay this morning, conveying a newly appointed Medical Commission of three or four of our resident doctors to visit the "Brisbane" in company with Dr Challinor, and determine whether she be admitted to pratique or not. These medical gentlemen are apparently to take a responsibility upon themselves in this particular instance, which properly belongs solely to the regularly appointed Health Officer, and which, until he is formally superseded, had, we think, be much better left in his hands. It is little more than forty-eight hours, since a Chinaman, sick with smallpox, was on board the "Brisbane", and our readers may, we think, form tolerably accurate opinions as to how far isolation of the patient could be practicable on board a steamer of 1700

> tons, carrying a numerous crew and 500 to 600 Chinese, in addition to saloon passengers and servants. A Governor or a Governor's servants are for anything we have ever heard to the contrary just as capable of carrying infection as less distinguished individuals, and therefore, if Sir Arthur Kennedy and his suite are exempted from the quarantine we shall have the questionable satisfaction of knowing that immigrants of less importance have been frequently imprisoned on Peel Island without cause, or else that a necessary law is to be set aside in this case with the concurrence of the Ministry, and for the personal convenience of the gentleman who is to become Her Majesty's representative. No one will be deceived concerning the creation of this special Medical Commission since there can only be one reason for the appointment. Had not Sir Arthur Kennedy been on board the "Brisbane" no Medical Commission would have been thought of, and the law would have been carried out as it has always been hitherto.

The medical commission duly visited the quarantined ship and after due consideration agreed with Dr Challinor, despite the fears expressed by the *Brisbane Courier*. A quarantine period of sixteen days from the date the patient was removed from the ship at Curtis Island was considered necessary. The saloon passengers and some remaining steerage passengers were transferred to the quarantine station on Peel Island. The government steamer *Kate* was hastily prepared to make it a suitable place in which the governor and his party could spend the quarantine period. And so, Miss Kennedy and her companion spent Easter cruising around Moreton Bay instead of enjoying the comforts of Government House as they had hoped. But their burden was lightened by the members of the Brisbane and Ipswich musical societies who went down the bay on Easter Monday night to give them a moonlight serenade concert from the deck of the *Lady Bowen* which had pulled alongside the governor's temporary steamer home. They were assisted in their efforts to entertain the viceregal party by Mr Harding, a pyrotechnic expert who arranged a grand display of fireworks.

On 10 April, the day the quarantine period would end, crowds of gaily dressed people flocked down Queen Street to the new Government Wharf at Petrie's Bight to welcome Sir Arthur. Such a gathering had not been seen in the colony since the visit of the Duke of Edinburgh some nine years previously. Probably the loyal people of the colony were anxious not only to welcome the new governor as their representative but also to express in this manner their sympathy for his enforced detention in the bay through the quarantine regulations. The governor was expected

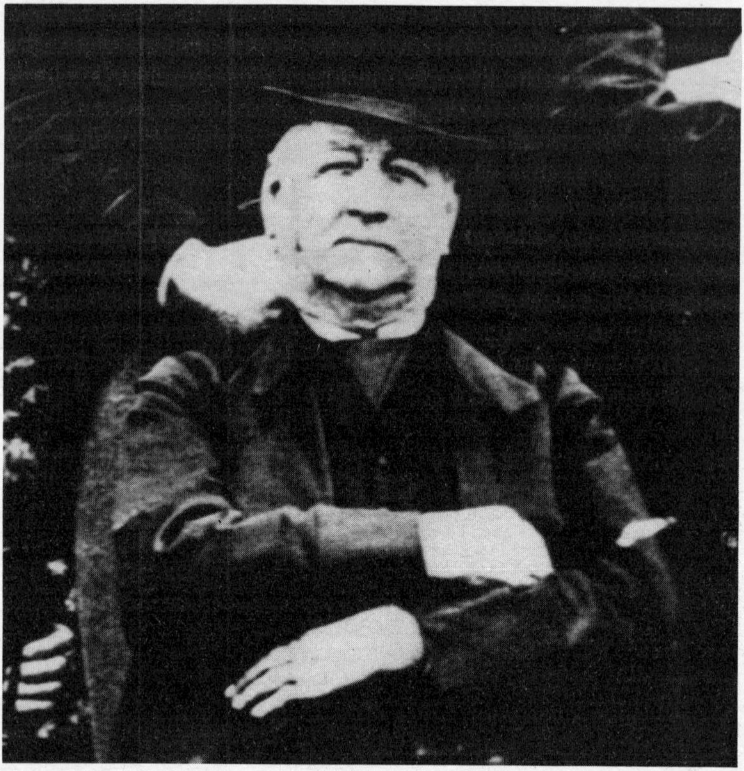

Sir Arthur Kennedy (around 1880). He was quarantined when he arrived to take up the position of governor of Queensland. (Courtesy Oxley Library)

at noon. The end of his quarantine was to be signalled by the firing of two guns and a blue flag would be hoisted on the Windmill Hill flagstaff when the steamer *Kate* was carrying him on his way to be greeted by his new subjects. But the crowd waited in vain for the sound of the guns. Anxious eyes turned towards Windmill Hill but no blue flag fluttered in the breeze. All kinds of rumours spread amongst the crowd. The governor had developed the disease; Miss Kennedy was nigh unto death; and so on. The truth was revealed the next day in this report in the *Brisbane Courier*.

> The Health Officer, Dr Challinor, boarded the "Kate" early yesterday morning, and before passing the vessel as free from infectious disease, proceeded in the usual manner for suspected smallpox, to submit all on board to a personal examination, including an inspection of the chest for any possible eruptions of the skin. Sir Arthur Kennedy sub-

mitted himself to this examination, but the ladies in the party made an objection in this case, which Sir Arthur strongly supported, and positively refused to allow the usual examination to be made. Dr Challinor, conceiving that his written instructions gave him no discretion for exceptional treatment, thereupon telegraphed to the Government in Brisbane that, not having been permitted to carry out his inspection in the way he thought necessary, he was unable to recommend the release of the "Kate" from quarantine. This message came before the cabinet at nine o'clock and Drs O'Doherty, Bancroft and Cannan, the gentlemen who formed the Medical Commission a fortnight since, to visit the steamer "Brisbane" and consult with Dr Challinor as to the advisibility of her being detained in quarantine, were on this second occasion called upon to perform a similar duty with regard to the "Kate". The gentlemen named at once obeyed the summons and in company with all the members of the Ministry proceeded as early as possible to the mouth of the river in the steamer "Laura". Dr Challinor came on board the "Laura" and held a consultation with the other medical gentlemen, who afterwards went aboard the "Kate", to make such inspection as they might [think] necessary. Sir Arthur Kennedy reiterated his objection and Dr O'Doherty stated that the Health Officer had no doubt acted consistently in accordance with with the letter of his instructions; it would be unwise in the present case to create a bad precedent, but he thought that the rule might with perfect safety be a little relaxed in this instance, as the ladies in question were blooming with health, and if they would expose their wrists he thought that would be sufficient. Drs Cannan and Bancroft concurred with this view and the request was promptly complied with. The doctors then returned to the "Laura" and reported to the Ministers (who were all present) to the effect that in their opinion the inspection made was all that was really required and the pratique might at once be granted with perfect safety. The Ministers held a cabinet meeting on board the "Laura", and in accordance with the recommendation of the Board ordered the "Kate" to haul down the yellow flag. Dr Challinor, however, refused his concurrence and put his protest in writing against the advice tendered by the Board. The Ministers afterwards all went on board the "Kate" and congratulated Sir Arthur and his party on the termination of their disagreeable detention on board ship. The "Kate" weighed anchor and steamed towards Brisbane with the "Laura" in company.

[There was some medical basis for O'Doherty's examination of the wrists only. Perhaps unwittingly, he was anticipating the future. In later years, when examination for suspected smallpox was still required, the forearms only were examined. The skin eruptions are most prevalent on the extremities in a person suffering from the disease.]

The long wait did not dampen the enthusiasm of the crowds assembled on the wharf and in Queen Street. Loud cheers rang out as the two gun signal was, at last, heard. They were repeated when the blue flag was hoisted on Windmill Hill. Around 3 o'clock, black smoke could be seen above Kangaroo Point and then the "Kate" with the "Laura" close behind, came into view. After the two vessels were made secure to the wharf, Sir Arthur Kennedy stepped ashore to pass through a guard of honour formed by members of the Queensland Volunteer Rifles, supported by an attachment of the mounted police. On a suitably decorated dais, addresses of welcome were delivered with an appropriate reply by the new governor. High above all, three Aborigines in ceremonial paint and armed with the traditional spear and nulla nulla looked on the scene with wonder. When the speeches were over, the bands of the Volunteer Rifles and the Brisbane Volunteer Fire Brigade played the national anthem. Sir Arthur Kennedy with his daughter stepped into a coach pulled by four grey horses. When other carriages carrying the premier and other dignitaries were assembled, the viceregal procession passed along Queen Street towards the Victoria Bridge to be greeted by dense crowds lining the route. At George Street, the cortege turned towards the domain and Government House. A week later, His Excellency gave prominent citizens an opportunity to pay their respects. In the published list of those who attended the names of Dr O'Doherty and Dr Cannan are included. The names of Dr Bancroft and Dr Challinor are missing. Perhaps both were busy with their professional duties.

Typhoid at Toowoomba

One of the most significant advances in medicine in the twentieth century has been the control of infectious diseases. In some cases this has been almost if not complete eradication. The various factors responsible include improved disposal of human wastes; chlorination of water supplies; pasteurization of milk; health education in general, and in particular in the preparation of food for infants; the use of effective immunizing agents; and treatment with new drugs. People living in Queensland in the nineteenth century faced life without these advances and suffered many epidemics. One disease which killed many was typhoid fever.

The day had not come when it was known that typhoid germs leave the body through the faeces and urine, and to infect a second person must be transferred to his food. The transfer takes place through flies, contaminated water and milk or the fingers of a carrier in food preparation. Outbreaks of the disease occurred on the goldfields and the railway construction camps. Of course, many towns did not escape the ravages of the disease which brought a heavy death toll. In 1878, one such town was Toowoomba, and the number of cases and deaths from the scourge so worried the authorities there that they petitioned the colonial secretary in Brisbane. As a consequence, the mayor of Toowoomba, John Garget, received a letter from the colonial secretary dated 26 April 1878, advising him that he and William Henry Groom, MLA for Drayton and Toowoomba, and Dr John Thomson, a prominent Brisbane medical practitioner, had been appointed a board, to find out why typhoid fever was so prevalent in Toowoomba, and also to find out how to suppress it.

The board went to work quickly. It made house-to-house inspections, including fifteen hotels and most of the business premises, and also visited all the public institutions, the Chinese gardens, the tanneries, and public baths. It considered that its duty "would not be complete without examining the medical gentlemen practising in the town". Their evidence was appended to the report, as was the evidence from the resident dispenser of the Toowoomba Hospital, the inspector of police, the inspector of nuisances and the nightman. By 6 May 1878, only eleven days after the date of the letter of appointment, the report was completed.

The board found that in the preceding four months forty-one deaths from typhoid fever and related diseases had occurred. These came from the town itself and in the areas adjacent.

Most of the seven hundred dwellings in the town had a cesspit and in approximately half, drinking water was obtained from a nearby well. In nearly every case the wells were situated about twenty feet away from the cesspits. The board devoted a special section of its report to this subject:

> CESSPOOLS
>
> These are an abomination, no matter they be roughly dug pits or well-cemented tanks. They are opposed to all hygienic rule. Surely no one can dispute that the sooner all excretions, whether solid or fluid, whether of men or of animals, are removed from around our dwellings, the better; and yet, instead of removing them or destroying them, we store them up, we hoard them as if they were treasures, and they putrefy and ferment, and a concentrated decoction percolates through the soil to contaminate our wells, while a poisonous gas is given off to pollute our atmosphere; and so, what between the water we drink and the air we breathe, we are charged with the germs of disease and death.
>
> This may seem absurd, and the question may be asked, "Why then do we not all suffer?" Man is a pliable and accommodating animal, and he can become accustomed to filth, just as he can to alcohol, tobacco, opium, or arsenic.
>
> It is admitted on all sides, that faecal matter becomes very much more dangerous after it under goes putrefactive change, and a great array of names can be brought forward to support the belief that typhoid fever can originate from the gases and matters generated during decomposition. If then the discharges of healthy subjects are productive of so much evil, how much greater must the danger be when the evacuations of typhoid patients, and the fluxes of those suffering from diarrhoea and dysentery, are stored up to rot and putrefy in our midst.

When it had inspected the business section of the town the board said:

> It might have been expected that public-houses, with their greater traffic, would have been most offensive, but in some instances they set a good example to the shops and warehouses.
>
> Banks and offices, which ought to have been clean, were, in some instances, conspicuous from presenting a very different appearance. And, with the exception of the Gaol, which was in perfect order, most of the other Government properties were in a very neglected condi-

> tion. The Immigration Depot was simply disgraceful. It is a tumble-down dwelling, quite unfit for the use to which it is put, but a little attention on the warder's part would prevent that dirt and neglect which was everywhere apparent . . .
>
> Sanitary arrangements [in the hospital are] very defective. There is a huge slop-pit of stagnant putrescence. This certainly is contrary to all notions of public health. Laundry water from the clothes of healthy persons is quite bad enough, but when from the garments and soiled bed-clothes of the diseased, it is infinitely worse. The water from the bath runs by open brick drain into James Street. Both dry-earth closet and the disused cesspit are in a most defective state.

A special section of the report was devoted to the Chinese gardens. It was believed that the gardeners used human wastes for fertilizer. The board considered that "these should be under the supervision of the Inspector, in order that any nuisances arising from the storage of ordure, or the manufacture of fluid manure, may be averted. The use of this fluid manure, made from cesspit contents, is attended with considerable danger to health. It is not trenched into the soil or poured around the roots of plants — it is rained over the plants themselves and its more solid particles may be swallowed with the blades of lettuce or of salad, if not cooked vegetables, such as cabbage, cauliflower, &c."

From the evidence of the inspector of nuisances for the municipality and the nightman it is seen that the city council, the corporation, did not operate a sanitary service for the residents. The inspector deposed that the closets were cleaned only under order from the council and there was no set period at which householders were obliged to empty them. Some closets were emptied twice a year, some only once, and some not so often. Some to his knowledge had not been emptied for three years. His statement was signed:

his
William X Thompson
mark

James Nathan, nightman and chimney sweep, said that emptying cesspits was purely a private arrangement. He made terms with the parties requiring his services. He used a horse and dray, with two casks, covered over with bags, to take the contents to a large hole in Queen's Park. There was no regulation which prevented him from selling or giving nightsoil away. But, he hastened to say, he had done this only twice and never to the Chinese gardeners.

The report stated: "It is quite unnecessary to argue whether for the production of typhoid, pre-existing typhoid has contaminated the water, or whether ordinary decomposing sewage in water is sufficient to produce the disease. Authorities are divided, and quite as many uphold the 'emanation' theory as uphold the 'transmission'. It will be sufficient if it be shown that the wells of Toowoomba are rendered impure by the admixture of sewage." Although these remarks show some confusion over how typhoid is spread, other statements in the report indicate that at least some of the factors which the board thought were responsible for the epidemic would still be acceptable when medical science later had shown beyond all doubt how the disease spreads. The causes of the prevalence of typhoid at Toowoomba were found to be drought, well water contamination, total neglect of ordinary cleanliness, and ignorance.

The Drought

The medical witnesses are of opinion that the continued dry weather was one of the causes of the prevalence of typhoid fever. The explanation of the theory is highly probable, and worthy of all credence. The wells at present are low from want of rain; the cesspits at present are full from carelessness and inattention. The ordinary soakage is not diluted as in times of plenty, but, owing to the scarcity of water, is highly concentrated and dangerous.

Well Water Contamination

That a majority of the wells of Toowoomba, and especially in Ruthven Street and surrounding neighbourhood, are contaminated by the introduction of sewage, there is every reason to believe, and none to doubt. It is the firm conviction of the medical witnesses, and it is the opinion of the few townspeople who very wisely have given up the use of well water and depend for their supply on other sources. It must surely be apparent to every one who has inspected the positions and contents of the wells and cesspits in Toowoomba. In fact, the relative situations of the two (wells and pits) make it imperative that there should be a connection between them, and it cannot be otherwise.

Total Neglect of Ordinary Cleanliness

It is hardly possible to imagine anything more filthy than the present condition of portions of Ruthven and Russell Streets. This does not refer to hygienic errors which require the services of a sanitary engineer to correct, but to the neglect of the ordinary precautions, not for the preservation of health only, but for the maintenance of common decency. Even simple tidiness, for the sake of outward appearance, is disregarded.

A most minute inspection of these streets revealed, in many places, little else than overflowing cesspits, filthy pig-styes, dirty poultry houses, offensive middens — sometimes dry, but more frequently wet, and consisting of every possible kind of refuse — putrefying accumulations of fruit and vegetables, ill-kept drains and stagnating slop-water and slime.

Ignorance

This has shown itself in the disposal of the evacuations from typhoid fever patients, and has contributed not only to the extension of the disease but to the increase of the death rate.

In a house some distance from the town (two miles), well ventilated and apparently free from all risk of the water being contaminated (the well is 115 feet deep) by the introduction of sewage, a case of typhoid fever occurred. That this was imported from town, where fever then existed, there is every reason to believe, for there is nothing at the house of the attacked to warrant the supposition that the disease could originate there "de novo".

The evacuations of this patient were, without disinfection or dessication, thrown into the common cesspit used by all the members of the family, and the effects of this were soon visible among others of the children who had not been exposed to the same risks, in town, as the first attacked. Four (4) suffered from typhoid and three (3) died and it was not until after the scourge had left the house that the father knew that if he had properly disinfected the discharges — covered them with dry earth and buried them somewhere in the paddock — the chances of contagion would have been very materially lessened, and, possibly, death prevented. A similar ignorance was displayed in other houses, and with the same lamentable results.

The board recommended several steps for the suppression and future prevention of typhoid fever in Toowoomba: the Proclamation of the district under the Health Act of 1872; the nomination of a medical gentleman, either as member or an officer of the local board of health, and the appointment of a qualified inspector; the total abolition of all cesspits; the substitution of the dry-earth system; the proper disposal of slopwater; the stopping of the present well-water supply, and the immediate use of reservoir water or rain water; the supervision of Chinese gardens; the banishment of all pigs from the municipality; the registration of disease; and the instruction of the young at school.

The 1872 Health Act came into force only when it was proclaimed for a particular area and the proclamation was only effective for six months. Under its provisions the muncipality was obliged to appoint a local health board which then had power to provide for the frequent cleansing of the streets; for the cleansing, purifying, ventilation and disinfection of houses, dwellings and other premises; for the removal of nuisances; for the prevention and mitigation of epidemic, endemic, or contagious disease; and for visiting and inspecting any dwelling or premises containing any filth or other matter dangerous to health, or where disease existed, or death had occurred. The board was enthusiastic concerning the use of dry earth to cover nightsoil. It said that "theoretically it is complete. Than dry earth nothing better can be had to destroy not only the contagion or infection of discharges, but the discharges themselves. It is the system sanctioned by the Mosaic law, as a reference to Deuteronomy, twenty-third chapter, thirteenth verse, will show; [And thou shall have a paddle upon thy weapon; and it shall be when thou wilt ease thyself abroad, thou shall dig therewith, and shall turn back and cover that which cometh from thee.] and it is in accordance with Nature, as the habits of the dog or cat can prove." Two of the recommendations were particularly interesting: whenever any contagious or infectious disease showed itself in a district or was developing, the medical attendant had to immediately report it to the local board of health, or to the proper authority, so that the necessary steps could be taken. The procedure became common practice in most developed countries but it was not until the 1900 Health Act was passed in Queensland that it became law. The board made the recommendation twenty-two years before. On the subject of health education in schools the board recommended that, "Children at the National or Grammar Schools should be taught the elements of physiology and the laws referring to public health, including the subjects of food, water, air, exercise, dress, ventilation, drainage, the dangers of excess or irregularity, and the absolute necessity of a most scrupulous cleanliness, not only as individuals, but in their houses, sheds, yards, drains, &C. as members of the community generally. Ignorance is at the root of a very great amount of the present sickness." In this recommendation the board was well ahead of its time.

Some of the board's recommendations were put into effect. The health act was proclaimed for the area and there was a move to use earth closets instead of cesspits. But the proclamation was not maintained and the community as a whole ignored most of the advice of the report. In 1883, Groom, who had now become mayor, persuaded the council to make efforts to do the work of the local board of health which had dissolved when the health act was no longer in force. He succeeded in having the necessary by-laws passed but when typhoid broke out again in 1884, and the by-laws had been confirmed by the colonial secretary, he sent this telegram on 28 April, to the colonial secretary.

> I regret to say that in consequence of the nonconfirmation of the bye-laws sent to the Colonial Secretary office in October and the withdrawal of the proclamation extending the Health Act to Toowoomba typhoid fever is again prevalent and the earth closets are in a most disgraceful condition. When will bye-laws be confirmed.
>
> W.H. Groom

The conditions prevailing in Toowoomba were typical of those existing in the whole of the colony. Contemporary reports reveal a similar picture in Brisbane. It was not until well into the twentieth century when the suggestions of the Toowoomba report and other improvements were effected that the disease became a rarity.

Too Drunk To Operate

Under the Crown Lands Alienation Act of 1868, large pastoral holdings in southeast Queensland were broken up and men took up smaller areas for agricultural purposes. In 1878, George Hope was farming on one of these selections near the tiny township of Nerang, some fifty miles south of Brisbane. A young Brisbane watchmaker, Alexander Youill, paid the Hope family a visit in May of that year. One evening, after an early meal, younger members of the family and employees were dancing to the strains of the accordion on the verandah of the farmhouse. As the dance livened up, the visitor from the city was dancing with the farmer's daughter, Mary. Suddenly, about 7 p.m., there was an explosion among the happy group. Youill fell to the floor, crying, "My leg, my leg!" Nearby lay a shot-gun, with the smell of gunpowder coming from its barrel. The brisker steps of the dancers had dislodged it from a nail on the verandah wall.

Youill was carried into the kitchen and his trouser leg was cut away. Blood was pouring from a large gaping wound in the calf of his left leg. A sheet was hastily torn to dress his wound and hopefully stem the flow of blood. He was then made as comfortable as possible on a bed. A farmhand rode to bring a neighbour. On his arrival, a conference was held to decide what was the best way of getting medical help for the wounded watchmaker. The nearest doctor was stationed at Beenleigh, thirty miles away on the track to Brisbane. It was agreed that the time a messenger would take to reach the town and return with the doctor would be longer than a journey to Brisbane with the injured man. The latter course was preferred but Hope had no suitable conveyance. The farmhand was again dispatched, this time to Nerang to borrow a spring-cart. It was 5 a.m. before the patient left the farm lying on a mattress on the floor of the uncovered cart. Neighbours on horseback, leading spare cart horses accompanied Hope who was in charge. The autumn sun was not hot, but the continual jolting as the cart passed over the rough track with many gully and creek crossings took heavy toll of poor Youill. The fifty-six miles to Brisbane took almost fifteen hours to cover and the hospital was reached at 8 p.m., twenty-five hours after the accident happened. Dr John Thomson, the house surgeon, examined a conscious but very weak patient. When he unwrapped the sheet bandages from the injured leg, he saw two broken bones, mangled muscles and tissues and a cold pulseless foot. He concluded that amputation was the only procedure.

In such circumstances, it was the house surgeon's duty to call one of the four honorary visiting surgeons who took it in turn to visit the hospital week about. As a telephone service in Brisbane was still two years away, Thomson called for his horse to be saddled and rode into Brisbane to consult Dr O'Doherty, who was the visiting surgeon for the week. He found him at home, in Harris Terrace, George Street, giving a dinner party. The guests included Dr Cannan, another visiting surgeon. O'Doherty instructed Thomson to call on the other two visiting surgeons to advise them that there would be a consultation on the case at the hospital at 10 p.m. This message was conveyed to Dr Mullen but the fourth visiting surgeon was out of town. Dr Mullen arrived at the hospital shortly after 10 p.m. but O'Doherty and Cannan came at 11.30 p.m.. Perhaps the dinner party delayed the two doctors but O'Doherty had made two house calls on the way. He had written a prescription for one patient.

At the consultation, the doctors all agreed that amputation was necessary. O'Doherty announced he would operate immediately and ordered the staff to have the patient and the operating theatre prepared. Then came a bombshell. Thomson told O'Doherty that he believed he was not in a fit condition to operate. With this Dr Mullen concurred. O'Doherty, usually noted for his genial nature, exploded, and his Irish temper flared. It was bad enough to be accused of such a condition but for the accusation to come from the house surgeon was bitter gall indeed. This was the beginning of several hours' wrangling, with poor Youill waiting ready for the operation. O'Doherty demanded of Thomson that he fetch Dr Hugh Bell, the consulting surgeon for the hospital and the hospital committee. Thomson refused, saying that Dr Bell seldom came to the hospital; the chairman was away and the other members of the committee were unlikely to come to the hospital at that hour of the night. At one stage, O'Doherty paced up and down on the hospital verandah, claiming later he did this so that he could not be accused of having gone to sleep off his debauch. At 1 a.m. Cannan left the hospital in a cab. At 2.30 a.m., Thomson at last decided to obey O'Doherty's instructions and again rode into town. When the house surgeon had not returned by 4 a.m. O'Doherty also left the hospital to walk back to his home in George Street. In Brunswick Street, he met Thomson returning to the hospital after consulting Dr Bell and Rev. Griffiths, one of the committee. Another bitter but briefer verbal exchange took place between the two, and each continued his way. At 6 a.m., thirty-five hours after Youill was shot, Dr Mullen, in the presence of Dr Bell, who had gone to the hospital, amputated Youill's leg above the knee. For two days the patient made satisfactory progress but then his condition deteriorated and he died four days after the operation.

The case attracted much attention in hospital, professional and political circles. The hospital committee held two special meetings on the subject. Unwisely, O'Doherty was not invited to

Dr John Thomson (around 1889). As a young house surgeon at the Brisbane Hospital, he was audacious enough to announce that the well-respected Dr O'Doherty was too drunk to operate. (Courtesy AMA Queensland branch)

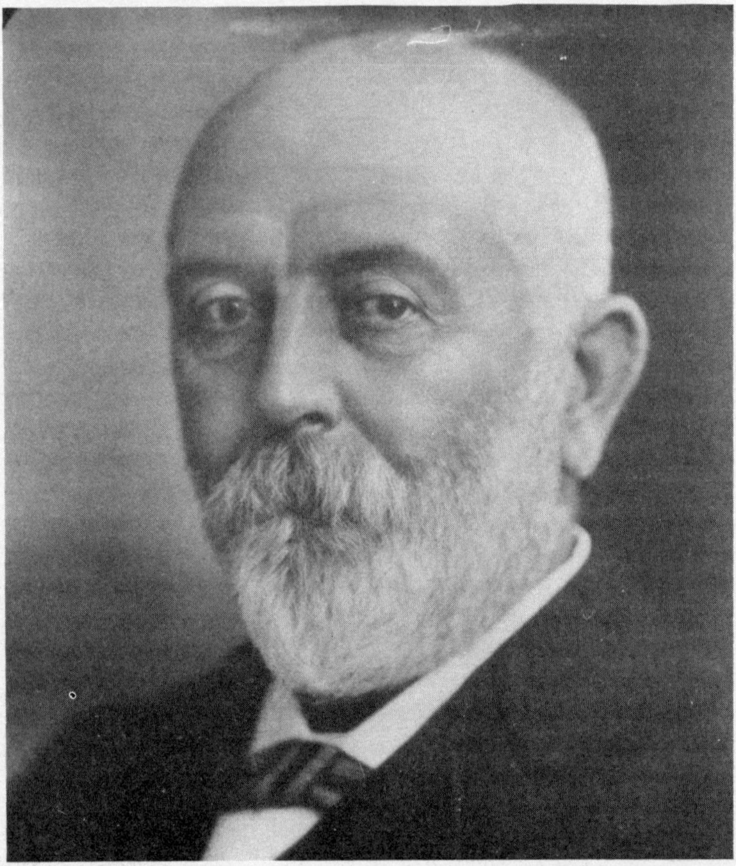

either of these although Doctors Mullen and Thomson were present. The first was held to examine the reason for the delay in the operation and the second to consider what action should be taken as a result of Youill's death. At the second meeting a letter from the Queensland premier, John Douglas, asking to be advised on the case, was read. Reports of both meetings appeared in the press. One report contained the following: "Other causes, which in the opinion of the committee it is not necessary here to record, and for which neither Dr Thomson nor Dr Mullen were in any way responsible, then delayed the operation." O'Doherty was condemned by implication. After the report of the second meeting appeared, O'Doherty refuted it in a letter published in the *Brisbane Courier*. He accused the committee of star chamber tactics in trying him in his absence and claimed it had shown great animus in hitting him below the belt. He referred to Thomson's claim that he was not fit to operate and said he had "indignantly repelled such an accusation, denied the right of the house surgeon, a paid officer, to sit in judgment on him and had requested absent staff members and members of the committee to be summoned to decide the matter". He pointed out that in the seventeen years he had been associated with the Ipswich and Brisbane hospitals he had performed almost every operation known in surgery and was quite willing to abide by the verdict of the public as to whether he had done his work creditably or not. He asked that the prescription that he had written just prior to his arrival at the hospital on the night in question be examined to determine whether any fault could be found in it.

At a subsequent magisterial enquiry, Thomson and Mullen reiterated that they had separately come to the opinion that due to certain circumstances O'Doherty should not operate on Youill. Both doctors were, however, emphatic that the delay in operating had not caused the death. They believed the poor condition of the patient brought on by the wound itself, the loss of blood and the exhausting journey from Nerang were the contributing factors. James Jackson, the chief wardsman, used less delicate language in his evidence. He said that O'Doherty and Cannan had arrived at the hospital the worse for drink and the patient had said that he would not allow O'Doherty to amputate his leg as he was too drunk. The magistrate apparently believed the medical evidence that the delay in operating had not caused Youill's death. In summing up, his main comments were a criticism of the carelessness of having a loaded gun in such a position that it could so easily be exploded.

At the first regular meeting of the hospital committee after the enquiry, O'Doherty again raised the subject, claiming that had Thomson summoned the consulting surgeon and the committee when he had first instructed him, the difficulty would not have arisen. The committee defended its condemnation of O'Doherty by implication by pointing out that not one word had been recorded in the minutes that the Irish doctor was at fault.

It is difficult to gauge what effect the episode had on O'Doherty's reputation. There is no doubt that he had antagonized the hospital committee and that there were people in the community who blamed him for Youill's death. Denis O'Donovan, the parliamentary librarian who was carrying on a vendetta against Bishop Quinn and his supporters, of whom O'Doherty was probably the staunchest, used the incident to tell Archbishop Vaughan in Sydney in a private letter that O'Doherty had been censured publicly for being drunk on duty. However, O'Doherty's standing in the community was so high at this time, that the incident would have been disregarded by most. From contemporary reports, it appears that he continued his many-sided career unaffected.

"Horsewhip the Doctor"

In the winter of 1890, a small group of Brisbane women prepared for the annual meeting of the Committee of the Hospital for Sick Children to be held on 16 July. Ever since the hospital, commonly known as the Children's Hospital, had been founded in 1878 by Mary McConnell in rented houses in Leichhardt Street, the affairs of the institution had been managed by a ladies committee with the help of a number of gentlemen who favoured the ladies with their opinion and advice. For a time the hospital was situated in Warren Street, Fortitude Valley, but in 1883, the hospital had shifted to Herston where a new building had been specially erected for the purpose with money raised by public subscription and government subsidy. The committee now realized that the building was inadequate but the colony of Queensland was entering on hard times and it was not opportune to ask for funds to replace it.

The year that had passed had been an eventful one. The committee had been saddened by the death of Alexander Archer and the loss of Mrs Lord in the wreck of the *Quetta*. They both had been ardent supporters of the hospital. But there had been bright spots also during the year. For the first time the nurses had been supplied with uniforms and visitors to the hospital had commented favourably on the neat appearance of the women who wore them.

The hospital had had the services of a full-time resident medical officer for twelve months, and the visiting medical staff were very satisfied with Alfred Jefferis Turner who had arrived just before the previous annual meeting to take the position. After the 1889 meeting, when Dr Turner moved through the people who had just attended the gathering, there were few who knew him. When the almost translucent little man was asked who he was he replied, "I am the new wesident medical officer". He had never been able to pronounce his Rs. The son of an English missionary to China, he had graduated from the London University College with the highest honours in 1884 and two years later had received a doctorate in medicine. He came to Queensland when it was suggested that the climate would benefit a suspected

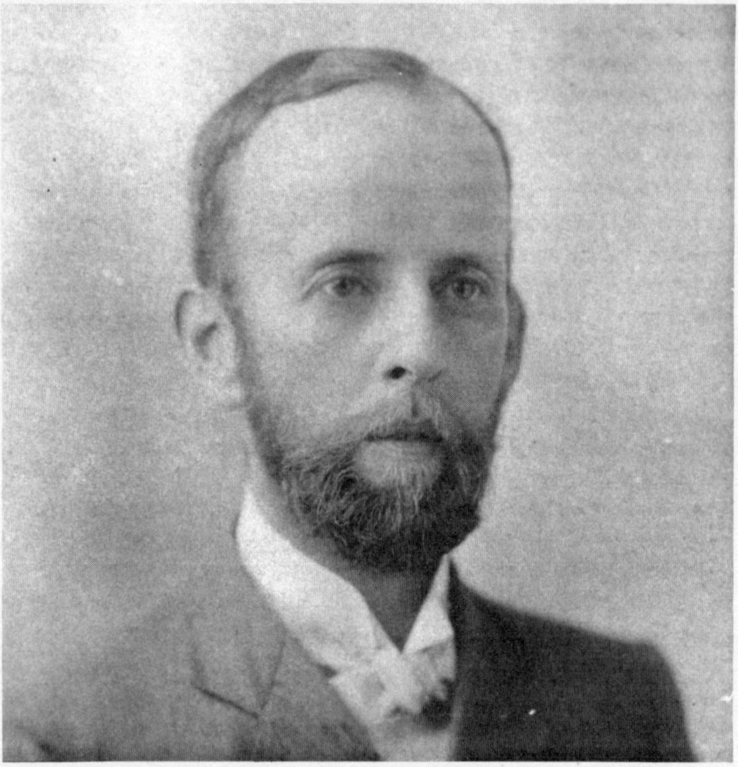

Dr A. Jefferis Turner in 1906, who with Dr Lockhart Gibson discovered lead poisoning in Queensland children. (Courtesy AMA Queensland branch)

infection of his lungs. In the year since his arrival, his mild manner, quiet voice, and kindness to his young patients won him the name of "Gentle Annie".

However, the ladies who assembled for the 1890 annual meeting were now looking on Dr Turner with some disfavour. It was true he had won approval for his work in the wards and for the first time an informative medical report was being presented for the annual meeting. But why, thought the ladies, had Dr Turner added the following report?

> Report upon the Defects of the Building and Site at present in use as a Hospital for Sick Children, in Herston Road, Brisbane.
>
> The present Hospital is a lofty, two-story building constructed entirely of wood, partly raised on piles, with the kitchen on the ground floor, and from its situation exposed to the winds from every quarter. Should a fire once get a hold on the building, (and this might occur at

any time) any attempt at extinction would be utterly futile, and the time available to clear the hospital of its inmates, even supposing there was no panic, would very probably be insufficient. The wards are already, in summer, full up to the limits of wholesomeness, and every available space is occupied.

The present accommodation for the nursing staff is insufficient and unsatisfactory. Not only is there no sitting or dining room for the nurses, but the matron's and nurses' bedrooms are separated from the wards only by thin wooden partitions, and all noises are heard in them as distinctly as in the wards themselves, so that sleep is often impossible.

Most of the wards are very draughty, and during the rainy weather much water gets into the wards in spite of all that has been done in the way of repairs. During the winter months cases of bronchitis contracted by children inside the Hospital are not uncommon. On the other hand one of the larger wards is, during the summer, so hot and close that it cannot then be used for bad cases, and is not well adapted for any.

There is no drainage system in the present building, but sewage matter is simply discharged down the hillside.

The ladies were surprised that such a nice young doctor had publicly condemned the building for which they had worked so hard. The rub was they knew he was correct. In a long and distinguished career that followed many more people were to be surprised at the criticism this seemingly mild retiring man would make. Many would know in their hearts that the criticism he made was generally correct. In 1894 the hospital committee approached the government for more level land nearer the adult hospital but the request was refused. Instead, the Diamantina Orphanage at South Brisbane was offered as a replacement for the Herston Hospital. The committee in turn rejected the proposal and in time the building Turner had justifiably condemned was replaced with a more substantial brick structure.

Turner graduated in medicine at a time when a new theory of the cause of infection was being hotly debated. In past centuries people believed that epidemics occurred because an angry god wished to punish the population for their sins. This belief was replaced by the miasmatic theory which was based on the concept that the infectious disease appeared when bad air or miasma resulted from certain climatic conditions and bad drainage. While Turner was growing up, a French scientist, Louis Pasteur, had demonstrated that infection was due to the invasion of specific germs. Like many men before him who introduced new concepts, Pasteur was ridiculed for his germ theory of disease. But

Pasteur's correct theory was accepted as, one by one, the organisms which caused the different diseases were isolated and identified. When Turner was in his final year before graduation, the organism that caused diphtheria was given the name of Klebs-Loeffler bacillus after the two men who had first discovered it. This was of vital importance to the medical world for the disease caused many deaths among children. It attacked first in the throat, often producing a murderous membrane which crept from the tonsils down the windpipe, suffocating the victim if an opening was not made and a tube inserted through which the little child could breathe. It was one of the cruellest diseases of the nursery. No wonder the Italians called it *garotillo* or the strangler. In Turner's first report he wrote:

> The diphtheria ward has been seldom empty many days together. During the last six months the cases have been of an unusually malignant character, and the mortality has been very high. It is usually the worst cases of this kind that are sent to hospital, often for the last resource of operative treatment. Altogether there have been 38 cases with 20 deaths. Two cases of slight membranous obstruction of the larynx recovered without operation, but it was necessary to perform tracheotomy in 21 cases and of these six lives were saved.

Apart from the operation to prevent suffocation there was no treatment for diphtheria at the time. In 1890, Turner commented, in the first of over a hundred papers on medical subjects he was to publish during his career, that he could not recommend enthusiastically any remedy, whether for internal administration or local application.

The high death rate from diphtheria continued and in 1894, Turner, now a visiting physician to the Children's Hospital, decided to go overseas to learn more about diphtheria and the new advances in the germ theory of diseases of which he was an ardent supporter. He went first to England, where he sadly informed his colleagues back in Queensland, very little important work in the field was being done. He then went to Germany, where he worked with two of the foremost medical scientists in the world, Robert Koch and Emil Von Behring. Von Behring was studying the poison that the diphtheria germ produced and which caused complications in parts of the body away from the throat. Sometimes the young patients developed heart conditions which resulted in heart failure and death. Sometimes the poison affected the nervous system. Von Behring found that when the poison was injected into horses the animals produced an antitoxin which could be used in the treatment of human patients with beneficial results. The German scientist was so impressed with the work of the doctor from Australia that he offered him a permanent position. Fortunately for Queensland and for Australia, Turner rejected the offer and returned to Brisbane. He immediately began using the diphtheria antitoxin in Brisbane, for there were still plenty of patients. He had remarkable success — in four years the mortality dropped from forty-two per cent to nine per cent. Whereas, before its introduction, almost every second person admitted to the hospital with diphtheria died, now fewer than one in ten patients died. Turner was keen to pass on to his colleagues what he had learnt in Germany. In a paper entitled "The Place of Bacteriology in Medicine" he pointed out that of all the cases admitted to the Children's Hospital since he came to Brisbane at least one-third suffered from diseases caused by germs that could be identified under the microscope. Of all the deaths, two-thirds came from these diseases. He said the profession could not afford to ignore the microscope and the new medical field of bacteriology. During the paper he spoke reverently of his "honoured teacher", Von Behring. He further warned his colleagues about claiming successful cures for diseases unless the diagnosis had been confirmed by isolating the organism.

While Turner was still a resident medical officer, he was treated as an equal by the visiting staff and friendships began that continued for years to come. The closest of these relationships was that which he developed with John Lockhart Gibson. Unlike Turner, Gibson was born in Queensland. He was the son of a Scot who managed the New South Wales bank at Ipswich. After attending Ipswich Grammar School, he went to Edinburgh, where, after a brilliant course he graduated in medicine in 1881. Returning to Queensland after lecturing in Edinburgh he was appointed a visiting physician to the Children's Hospital in 1888. Gibson later restricted his practice to eye diseases. The collaboration between Gibson and Turner began in 1892 when two young sisters from Cairns were admitted to the hospital in Brisbane. Their main clinical sign was a severe anaemia and their mother volunteered the information that each girl had a fascination with playing in dirt. In a brilliant cooperative effort the two doctors diagnosed the first cases of hookworm to be reported in children in Australia. The hookworm larva enters the body through the skin from contact with soil which has been contaminated with the eggs of the worm passed out through the faeces. The diagnosis

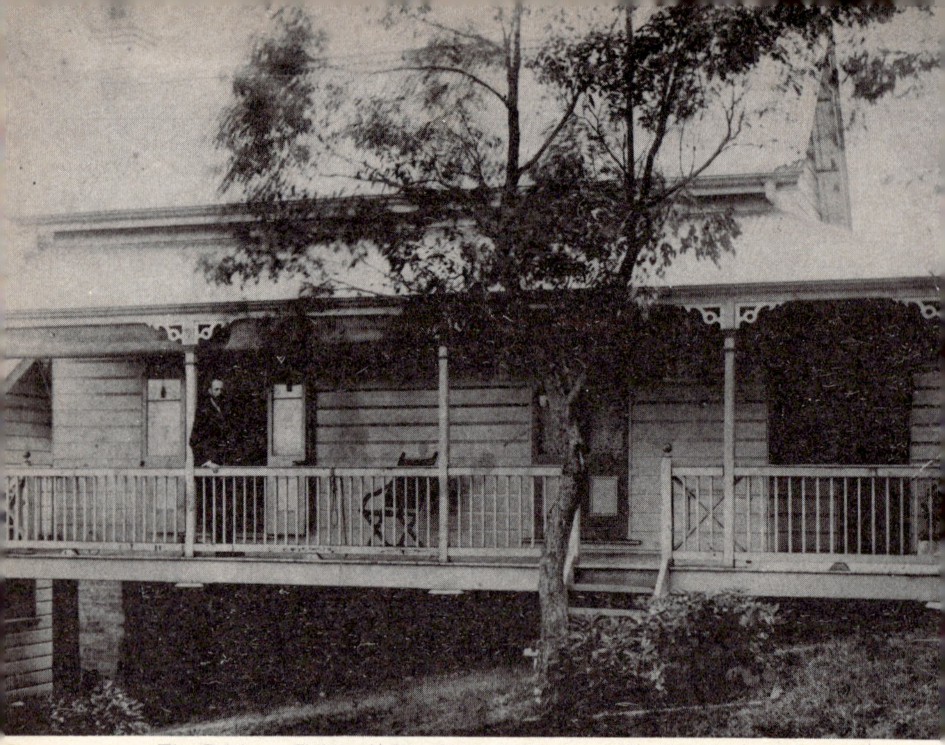

The Brisbane Children's Hospital built this house for the first resident medical officer, Dr A. Jefferis Turner (pictured around 1889), in the hospital grounds at Herston. (Courtesy Oxley Library)

The diphtheria ward at the Brisbane Children's Hospital, Herston, around 1899. Here Dr Turner administered the first anti-toxin in 1895. (Courtesy Oxley Library)

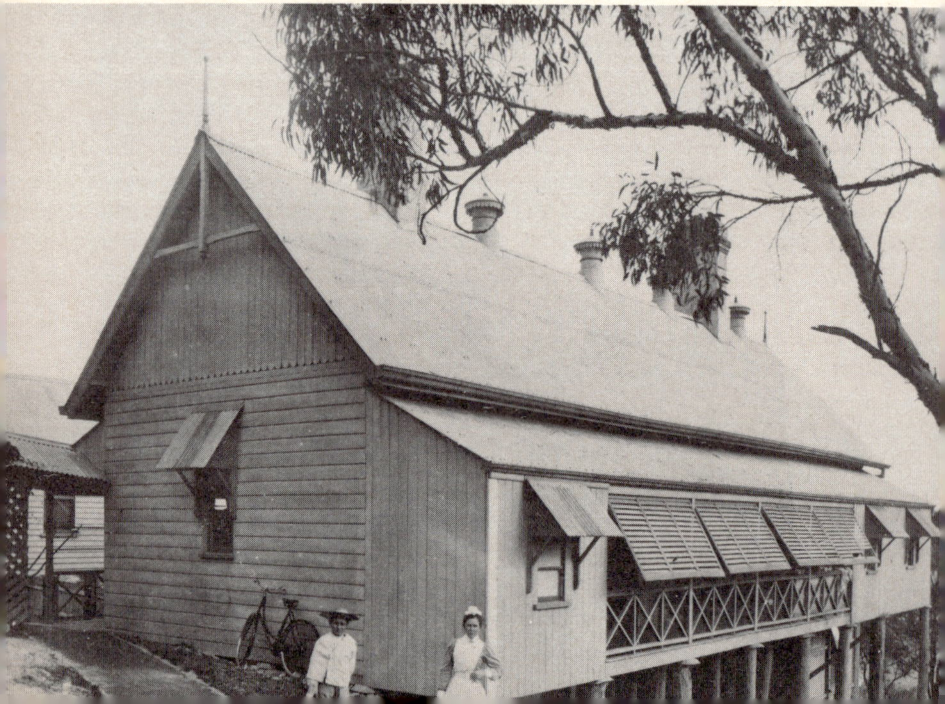

was confirmed by Gibson and Turner who identified the eggs of the hookworm in a microscope. The two collaborators illustrated a significant paper — which was read at the Intercolonial Medical Congress held in Sydney — with pen and ink drawings of the hookworm eggs. Further cases were found and in the years that followed Turner fought a campaign against the widespread scourge. Realizing the need for health education, he prepared a pamphlet describing the disease and how it could be prevented. Copies of the pamphlet were sent by Turner to every centre from which a case came to the Children's Hospital. His one-man fight against the disease met with little success. Frustrated by the inaction of the government and local authorities, in 1909 he published a statement which said: "When our statesmen have a little time for things that really matter, I should like them to pay some attention to the ravages of parasitic anaemia." Even this criticism did not arouse officialdom and it was not until 1917 when the Rockefeller Foundation in America sent a team to Queensland that something was done about the disease.

But it was their efforts with another disease that the names of Turner and Gibson are more often associated in Queensland's medical history — lead poisoning in children. The story began in 1890 and extended over thirty years. It is a story of astute clinical acumen; of a persistence necessary to convince sceptical colleagues; of a search for the source of the trouble and of a long battle to persuade politicians to legislate to remove the cause. It is difficult to apportion credit. Throughout the long years that the dramatic tale was unfolding the two men were in close and friendly collaboration. They would not have wished the tale to be told in any other manner.

There are many ill-effects of chronic lead poisoning — paralysis, damage to the red blood cells, blindness, and swelling of the brain which may progress to coma and death. Turner saw the first case six months after he arrived in Brisbane and while he was still the resident medical officer at the hospital. Writing later, he frankly admitted that he attributed the paralysis that occurred to another disease from which there was no hope of recovery. It was only when the young patient improved that he thought of lead poisoning. When further cases were admitted with an inability to raise the foot and/or straighten the wrist he suggested the diagnosis to Gibson who agreed with his resident medical officer. Gibson demonstrated the case before members of the Queensland Medical Society. Many doubted the opinion expressed by the two doctors that the illnesses were due to lead poisoning. Now confining his practice mostly to eye disease, Gibson found many patients in whom he believed eye conditions were the result of lead poisoning. Colleagues at the Children's Hospital gradually accepted the diagnosis. At the Intercolonial Medical Congress in Sydney, the honorary visiting medical staff and the resident surgeon of the Brisbane Children's Hospital were joint authors of a paper recording "a disease of children not previously recognized in Australia". Wilton Love, David Hardie and Peter Bancroft combined with Turner and Gibson to tell doctors from all states and New Zealand how lead poisoning was affecting some of Queensland's young population.

As Queensland doctors became more aware of the possibility of lead poisoning more cases were reported. There was no doubt, at least in Queensland, that the condition was a definite threat to the health of children, and the medical profession saw the urgency of discovering how the lead got into the bodies of the young patients. There were many suggestions: lead in the "silver" paper in which sweets were wrapped; lead found by analysis of some specimens of ginger beer; solder in tinned jams and galvanized tanks. One by one, the suggestions were ruled out by Brownlie Henderson, the government analyst, who, however, confirmed the diagnosis by finding lead in the urine of the patients. Still worried, in 1897 Turner said this in one of his many papers on the subject:

> Children in Queensland are suffering in no small number from a preventable form of poisoning. All I wish to prove is that a case has been made out for enquiry into its causation. The most essential part of this enquiry will be the co-operation of a chemical expert, for this is really a chemical problem. The medical expert has done his part if he points out that the poisoning exists, and where it exists. Furthermore, he is entitled, I think, not as an expert but as a citizen, to ask that the matter be investigated, that this large amount of suffering, disablement, blindness and death be put an end to.

The Queensland government responded by appointing a royal commission, comprising William Taylor, member of the upper house of parliament and eye specialist, Sandford Jackson, medical superintendent of the Brisbane Hospital and Wilton Love, visiting physician to the Children's Hospital and secretary of the Central Board of Health, to investigate the problem. For some reason the enquiry was terminated by the politicians before much work had been accomplished. Efforts to continue the investigation were in vain and the mystery was unsolved for the time being.

It was Gibson who came up with the solution in 1904. While sitting on his verandah one Sunday afternoon thinking about the subject, he suddenly arose and wiped the verandah rails with a linen cloth. Taking it to Henderson, the analyst, he asked him to look for soluble lead in the powdered paint that he had wiped up with the cloth. Henderson found plenty of lead in the sample. Later that week, Gibson suggested the possibility of powdered paint being the source of the lead to the mother of two patients he was treating. She told the eye specialist that the two patients were the only members of her family who bit their nails. At the time, most Queensland houses were built of wood and the hot sun soon reduced to powder the paint with which they were covered. Children playing on verandahs often rubbed their hands on verandah rails covered with powdered paint containing lead. Further questioning of patients suffering from the condition revealed that all had been exposed to the risk of swallowing lead in powdered paint. Most of these children either sucked their fingers or bit their nails.

Convinced they were correct, the two doctors now began a campaign to have the source removed. Their aim was to have the paint used on surfaces to which children would be exposed contain little or no lead. The battle lasted for years. The doctors were supported by the Queensland branch of the British Medical Association and the Intercolonial Medical Congress. They were opposed by the master painters. At last, in 1922, the Health Act was amended to demand that paint used on surfaces to which children would be exposed contain no more than five per cent of soluble lead. In another chapter of the lead poisoning story doctors found that another ill-effect of lead intake was the development of chronic kidney disease. In 1955, the act was again amended to prohibit the presence of lead in paint completely — more than fifty years after lead in paint was found to be dangerous.

In 1900 Turner was involved in another incident which revealed his fearlessness. In that year bubonic plague — the Black Death of Europe in centuries past — came to Queensland. The disease is transferred to man from infected rats by the bites of fleas. Prevention consists of the destruction of all rats and their breeding places as well as the elimination of food scraps left carelessly about on which the animals may feed. When the disease was reported from Townsville and Rockhampton, Turner volunteered to go north and help in the campaign to eradicate the scourge by acting as bacteriologist and health officer. Turner described the conditions he found at Townsville:

> The plague hospital was six miles out of town, and but for me would have been placed much further out. In those days there were no motor cars. The town was in a very insanitary condition. The stenches in the main street were worse than any I had encountered since I visited the Chinese city of Shanghai. Every vacant allotment was covered with rubbish affording splendid cover for rats. There was no provision for the collection of kitchen refuse and rat food was easily obtainable. On the town common, I counted eighteen rotten horse carcasses. This, I told them, was not the way to sweeten the sea breezes.

After three weeks of urging the Townsville council to begin a war on rats, no action had been taken. Turner sent a written statement to the municipal fathers which was published in the *Townsville Bulletin*.

> Sirs,
>
> As you are doubtless already informed, a case of plague has occurred in the centre of the city. . . When the plague once reaches a city it usually remains there several months, and the city of Townsville must not expect to be an exception. Whether you will have only a few cases of the disease during this time, or whether you will have many cases with a large mortality, depends certainly on yourselves.
>
> At present the sanitary condition of your city is bad, and you are not making haste to improve it. I have now been here over three weeks, and, although I must acknowledge the courtesy with which I have been formally accepted, I cannot see that anything has been actually done. I recommended the wholesale poisoning of rats; so far not one single rat has been poisoned by the Municipality. I advised the distribution of leaflets to householders. I am informed that these have been printed, but not yet distributed. I earnestly advocated the clearing of the city of rubbish. I am not aware that a single cart-load has yet been removed as a result of my representation. The Municipality of Cairns did more in the three days I was there than the Municipality of Townsville has effected in three weeks.
>
> You have an able and energetic Health Officer in the person of Dr. Linford Row. I have asked for his correspondence book, and find that he has given you most excellent advice, which you have not taken.

The mayor, Alderman McCreedy, was furious. At a public meeting he said Turner had greatly overstated the case. He claimed that Townsville was the cleanest city in north Queensland. Alderman Smyth claimed Turner had been given three days in Brisbane to examine plague and had come north as an expert. Little did the alderman know of the training that the doctor had undergone in Von Behring's laboratory in Germany. One speaker accused Turner of insulting the living and desecrating the dead. Another declared that the doctor should be horsewhipped for defaming Townsville. But Aldermen Blakey and Foley supported the visitor and finally convinced their colleagues that action was necessary. The city fathers started by burning the house in which the last plague victim had lived.

Turner now became more interested in the preventive side of medicine. Going overseas in 1901, he studied public health at the Guy's Hospital Medical School in London. The Queensland government took advantage of his presence in England and he represented the state at the International Conference for the Prevention of Tuberculosis. Tuberculosis was the leading cause of death in Queensland, killing over four hundred of the state's population of less than half a million each year. Most victims were in the prime of life. Turner's report on his return summarized the position in Queensland, and noted the recommendations from the conference, of which the main point was treatment of those in the curable stage of the disease in sanitaria. Turner outlined three parts of this type of cure: "life absolutely in fresh air, good feeding and exercise graduated to the individual needs of each case". Open-air wards with roll-up canvas blinds were erected at the Diamantina Hospital. They met the needs of fresh air treatment but were very uncomfortable in wet weather.

Shortly after his return from England, Turner, along with a number of other Queensland doctors, bought one of the early motor cars seen in Brisbane. As it rattled over the rough Brisbane streets, people noticed that the doctor had attached a large piece of hessian to the undersurface of the vehicle. One story has it that the hessian caught the nuts that fell off. Another says that it protected the undercarriage from the sticks and stones that flew up from the road's uneven surface.

Turner became a leader of his profession and highly respected not only in Queensland but also in other Australian states and in New Zealand. He was chairman of the children's section of the Australasian Medical Congress in Melbourne in 1908 and again in New Zealand in 1927. A guardian of high professional standards, he chose for his presidential address to the Queensland branch of the British Medical Association in 1907, the title, "The Medical Ideal"

If I had to classify the men I know, I should do so according to their

> ideals. Similarly, I would classify the professions according to their ethical ideals. Why should the ethical standard of the medical man be higher and more exacting than that of tradesmen? It is not because medical men, as individuals, are ethically superior to tradesmen. The distinction lies in the nature of the profession itself. When buying a pound of tea from the grocer, the purchaser can assess the quality. The purchaser of medical advice is no competent judge of the advice he purchases, although he may think he is. It is part of the medical ideal that a practitioner having once undertaken a case, whether for a large fee or a small one or for no fee at all, must do absolutely his very best for his patient. There are no limitations. He is bound to treat his lodge patients and his private patients with equal care, skill and attention. Success in the practice of medicine is not to be measured by the extent of a man's income.

Later generations will probably sneer at these remarks. However, Turner's beliefs in regard to professional conduct won for the medical profession the high image that it held.

When Jefferis Turner came to Queensland in 1889, every sixth baby born in Brisbane died before it reached its first birthday. In the inner suburbs the infant mortality was even higher. Many babies died from ignorance — ignorance on the part of the mother, but often ignorance on the part of the doctor also. Writing later with great humility, Turner talked of his own lack of knowledge on the subject but he made a special effort to overcome his deficiency.

> When I started private practice this baby problem obsessed me. Only then did I realise my own ignorance. I sought guidance from all the latest books. Among them was one that came from New Zealand on the feeding and care of the infant. This taught me much, though I did not agree with all it contained. I procured accurate scales and weighed every baby at every opportunity. I tried many methods of feeding and made appalling mistakes. I gained knowledge slowly, but it was based on hard experience. After a few years I began to enquire into the causation. Why were those babies being artificially fed? I found that in about every case that they had been weaned for no good reason.

The bottle-fed babies had by far the higher mortality. Gastroenteritis from infection of the baby's feed was responsible for many deaths. Turner advocated breast feeding but realized in some cases this was impracticable. He then joined with others in endeavouring to supply safe milk for Brisbane infants. The Lady Chelmsford Milk Institute was established in 1908 and began providing pasteurized milk. However, the project failed as the result of technical and distribution difficulties. During the period it operated Turner gave his services to the first baby clinic in

Queensland. In a paper he delivered in 1910 on *Infant Mortality* he said that the factors influencing his infant mortality were social, economic and moral as well as strictly medical. In suggesting a moral factor, Turner was thinking of how illegitimate babies were greatly disadvantaged and poorly cared for. The answer did not lie in any medical advances but in education of the mothers. The press took up the campaign in articles with headlines such as "The Cry of The Children" and pressed the government for infant welfare services. Women's organizations joined in deputations to wait on the home secretary but nothing had happened by the time that World War I broke out.

In the shortage of resident medical officers which that conflict brought, Turner, along with Lilian Cooper, returned to the hospital as house officer. In 1916 patriotism stirred him. He went to England and, at the age of fifty-five, joined the Royal Army Medical Corps. When he returned to Brisbane he found that the government had at last acted and four baby clinics were functioning, at Fortitude Valley, Woolloongabba, West End and Spring Hill. Although there was no medical director, Florence Chatfield, matron of the Diamantina Hospital, had been appointed part-time nursing supervisor. Turner resumed his former position of visiting medical officer to that hospital and when he had attended to his duties in the tuberculosis wards he discussed infant welfare

Dr and Mrs Turner in their De Dion Bouton in 1904. (Courtesy Oxley Library)

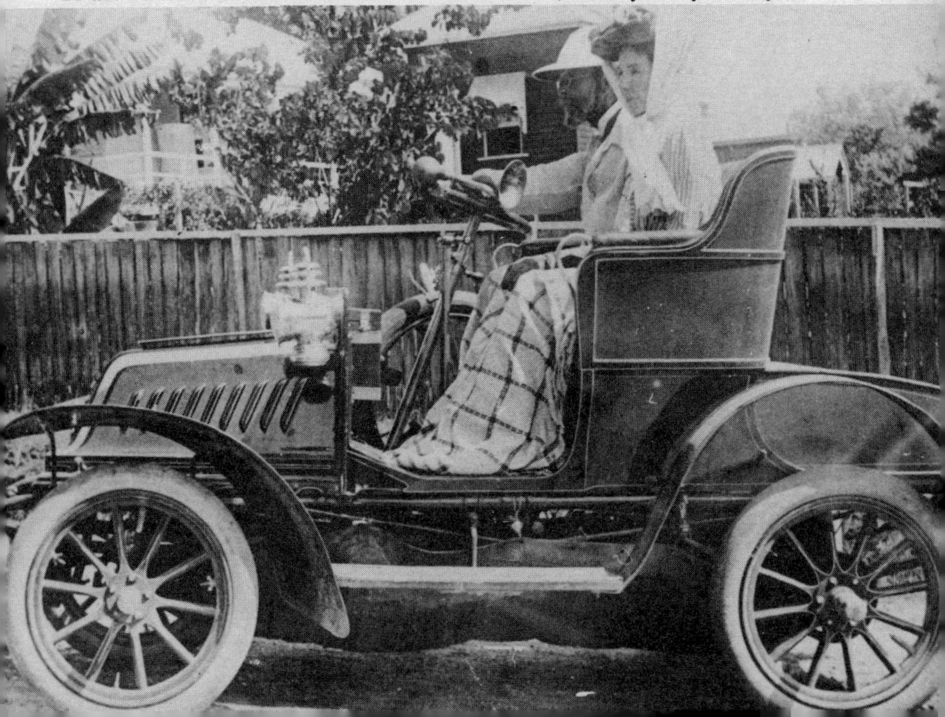

with Miss Chatfield. He thus became an unofficial adviser to the service. In 1922 Turner was appointed honorary medical officer to the Valley clinic. Then, in 1926, at the age of sixty-five, when most men are thinking of retiring, the energetic doctor became part-time director of the whole Infant Welfare Service. It was the beginning of eleven years of earnest endeavour to lower infant and maternal mortality in Queensland. Soon after he took up duty he visited all the clinics in the state. He was pleased with the work of the sisters but disappointed with certain aspects of the service. The service was not well known and when it was, its purpose was misunderstood. The relationship between the clinic sisters and members of the medical profession was poor and that with the staff of maternity hospitals was even worse. Turner began a publicity campaign. He called on all the doctors individually and lectured to them in groups despite his quaint lisp. Wherever he could, he talked to women's organizations. Although sometimes poorly attended, his lectures were often fully reported in the press. Lecturers from maternity hospitals began attending full courses in infant welfare.

He attended the Australasian Medical Congress in New Zealand in 1927, to chair the children's diseases section. New Zealand had for years a better record in the field of infant mortality than Australia. Their infant care was influenced by Sir Truby King with whom Turner did not always agree on the subject in which they were both regarded as experts. Their debates were vigorous but amicable.

Returning to Australia he began to expand the service. Despite the difficult financial period that the state was experiencing new clinics were opened and a child welfare rail clinic was commissioned to travel those parts of the state in which clinics were as yet not functioning. Every opportunity was taken to educate the expectant and nursing mother. Besides the important face-to-face instruction at clinic attendances the radio, newspapers, books and pamphlets were used. Much of the information contained in pamphlets issued by the service was later published in the popular *Queensland Mothers Book.* When Turner retired at the age of seventy-six, the clinics had increased from sixteen to eighty and the infant mortality had decreased from fifty deaths per every one thousand births to thirty-six. Of course, not all of this reduction can be attributed to the Infant Welfare Service but it played a very important role.

In a full and productive medical career in which this energetic man was active for a decade longer than most, Jefferis Turner was involved in many different aspects of the profession — clinical work, public health and preventive medicine, professional leadership, medical politics and the lobbying of parliamentarians on important medical issues. It was surely enough for one man. But, all the time, he was engaged in a separate field.

He was an amateur naturalist and contributed greatly to our knowledge of various subjects in this field. Here again, he appeared to be two men. Out in the field wearing his pith helmet and carrying his butterfly net, he looked like the original model for the caricatures so often depicted. One tale reveals this side of his naturalist's activity. Waiting one night on a suburban railway station, he noticed an uncommon moth fluttering around the light up a pole. The agile little man climbed the pole to catch the insect. His actions attracted many onlookers. Talking about the incident later, he said in his quaint language, "I was after a ware moth. When I got down, there was a quite a cwowd".

He collected extensively throughout Australia and his valuable collection of over fifty thousand specimens was bequeathed to the museum of economic entomology of the Council of Scientific and Industrial Research (now the Commonwealth Scientific and Industrial Research Organisation) in Canberra. However, he was far more than a mere collector. Ian Mackerras, director of the Queensland Medical Research Institute, wrote the following in an obituary.

> He gave to entomology more than could be reasonably expected of one man devoting his whole life to the subject. His work was by no means superficial. He was not content with simple descriptions of new species, merely adding hundreds of names to the list for others to elucidate later; he was actively concerned with evolution and classification, with orderly and systematic presentation of the knowledge he acquired, and he brought an extremely clear, logical and judicial mind to his work.

He contributed over a hundred papers or more to reputable scientific journals. Many are regarded as extremely valuable additions to the store of knowledge in this field.

"Gentle Annie" died at his Highgate Hill home at the age of eighty-six. His last official publication was an obituary for his collaborator and life-long friend, John Lockhart Gibson. One wonders how he found time to contribute so much in not one field but two fields of endeavour. He was small in physical stature but he stands out like a giant in the pages of Queensland's medical history.

Leper Islands of Moreton Bay

For centuries the cry of the leper was heard in many countries. The treatment meted out to the unfortunates who suffered from the disease was based on advice given in biblical times.

> The Lord spake unto Moses and Aaron, saying. . . "And the leper in whom the plague is, his clothes shall be rent, and his head bare, and he shall put a covering upon his upper lip and shall cry, Unclean, unclean.
>
> "All the days wherein the plague shall be in him he shall be defiled: he shall dwell alone; without the camp shall his habitation be."

For a long time these methods of control failed to eradicate the disease and it persisted in many parts of the world. However, harsh methods produced the desired effect in Europe by the end of the sixteenth century. Lepers were virtually entombed in lazarettos. When they ventured out they dressed in a way that denoted their disease. They rang a bell or sounded a rattle to warn the healthy that they were coming. These rules brought results and the disease died out.

When Britain decided to establish a convict settlement in Australia, she had been free of leprosy for three centuries. For this reason, the doctors of early Queensland, unfamiliar with the disease, failed to recognize it when it appeared in their patients — patients who came, not from Europe, but from China and the Pacific Islands. The Brisbane Hospital records of 1855 contain the following clinical notes of a Chinese, Oun Tsar.

> Had some disease of the first toe of left foot — it has been removed and there is now an opening into the head of the great toe of the same foot from which there is a slight foetid discharge and a probe detects loose bone. The last phalanx of the second finger of the right hand and soft parts have sloughed away.

There is no mention of a diagnosis of leprosy in the records but the description fits the disease. Joseph Bancroft, eminent physician and medical researcher, frankly admitted that many cases of "Islanders Toe Disease" that he saw were undoubtedly suffering from leprosy but that he failed to diagnose them as such when he was superintendent of the Brisbane Hospital in the late 1860s.

Reports of the disease among the Chinese and the South Sea Islanders continued with an odd case appearing among Europeans who had contracted the infection outside the colony. A German who worked as a wardsman at the Brisbane Hospital was exposed to leprosy in the Sandwich Islands and showed the telltale signs of the disease after he arrived in Queensland. A grave digger in a inland town and a sugar plantation worker in the north were reported as lepers. These cases were followed by the appearance of leprosy in the Aborigines.

The government deported a few Chinese with the disease but no real action was taken until around 1890. A leper station was established at Cooktown where a few Chinese patients were segregated in 1889. These were later transferred to Dayman Island twelve miles southwest of Cape York and then to Friday Island where they were supervised by Arthur Salter, medical officer to the cottage hospital on Thursday Island. The government was stirred into real action when the first case of leprosy appeared in a white patient who had spent all his life in the colony. He was a young man named Quigley living at Rockhampton. He was transferred to Brisbane where he was isolated in a tent at the Brisbane Hospital. From there he was taken to Stradbroke Island. The following extract is taken from an account written by a *Brisbane Courier* reporter accompanying the colonial secretary, Horace Tozer, who made a special trip on 12 April 1892 to see Quigley.

> The principal object of the Colonial Secretary's visit to Dunwich, however, was to inspect the leper station and to interview Quigley, the leper from Rockhampton. The station is distant two miles from the Dunwich Benevolent Asylum situated on the crest of a hill which slopes right down to the water's edge. The view from the verandah of the cottage is sublime and full of glorious colouring. The waters of the Bay stretch away to the horizon, ever flashing and changing, now green, now golden, now blue, now silver, as the clouds cross the sun, and shade and light chase each other. The islands are numerous and their green foliage can be distinctly observed, while the shores are lapped by the restless waves. Away to the right is a charming loch, the waters of which glint and sparkle like a sea of silver. It is altogether an enchanting spot, and it is hard to believe that amidst it all and close to where we stand is the foul blot of leprosy. Quigley himself greets us with a half-shy smile; he has a hammer in his hand, his sleeves are rolled up, and it is evident that he has been at work. He informs us that he has taken possession of his new home and is engaged in putting things straight. He is a tall slim youth, with the marks of leprosy on his hands and ears, and also on the nasal organ.

One wonders whether Quigley, cut off from civilization in the prime of life and facing an almost certain slow lingering death from a horrible disease, shared the reporter's enthusiasm for the beauty of his surroundings.

After the government had segregated these early lepers it began to have doubts about its power to do so. It accordingly passed the Leprosy Act of 1892 which provided for the proclamation of certain areas as lazarets and the detention of sufferers. The attitude to the disease at this time is reflected in the speech of the colonial secretary, Horace Tozer, in introducing the legislation.

> It is usually admitted at the present time that it is only by segregation — which is the principle of the Bill — that any community can rid itself of this loathsome, repulsive and unclean disease. I am informed that under clean and hygienic surroundings, wholesome diet and intelligent medical treatment, the separation will hardly be felt — and in the latter stages of the disease they are only too glad to hide themselves — and their lives will be naturally prolonged. This is the humane provision of the Bill.

Hansard also records another speech by the member for Croydon, Mr Hoolan, who pointed out the difficulties in making an accurate diagnosis of leprosy:

> Mr Hoolan said he had a little experience of the difficulty of detecting leprosy, as he was present at the medical examination of a Chinese leper some few years ago. What he saw there bore the contention that it was a very difficult matter to pronounce judgment on a case of leprosy, and with most doctors it was merely guesswork. Some four years ago a Chinese leper was discovered at Georgetown. The inhabitants said he was a leper, and refused to have any dealings with him. He got away from Georgetown, as he thought the police were going to shoot him and went to Croydon. The police magistrate at Croydon, Mr Cusack, got notice of the matter, and the police took charge of the man. A medical examination was made of the man by Dr O'Doherty, and there were also present Dr Freeman, Dr Flood, Mr Cusack and himself. Dr O'Doherty, after examining the man closely, said that his was a true case of leprosy; Dr Freeman said the case was a pronounced case of leprosy in a bad stage, and Dr Flood admitted that he had had no previous experience of leprosy, but thought from all he had heard and read that the case was a bad case of leprosy. Then Mr Cusack examined the man, but not from a medical point of view, and perhaps his examination was as skilful as the medical examination. He examined the man with the end of a walking stick and touched his sores and swelling. He decided that it was not a case of leprosy and the man was set at large. It would be a deplorable state of

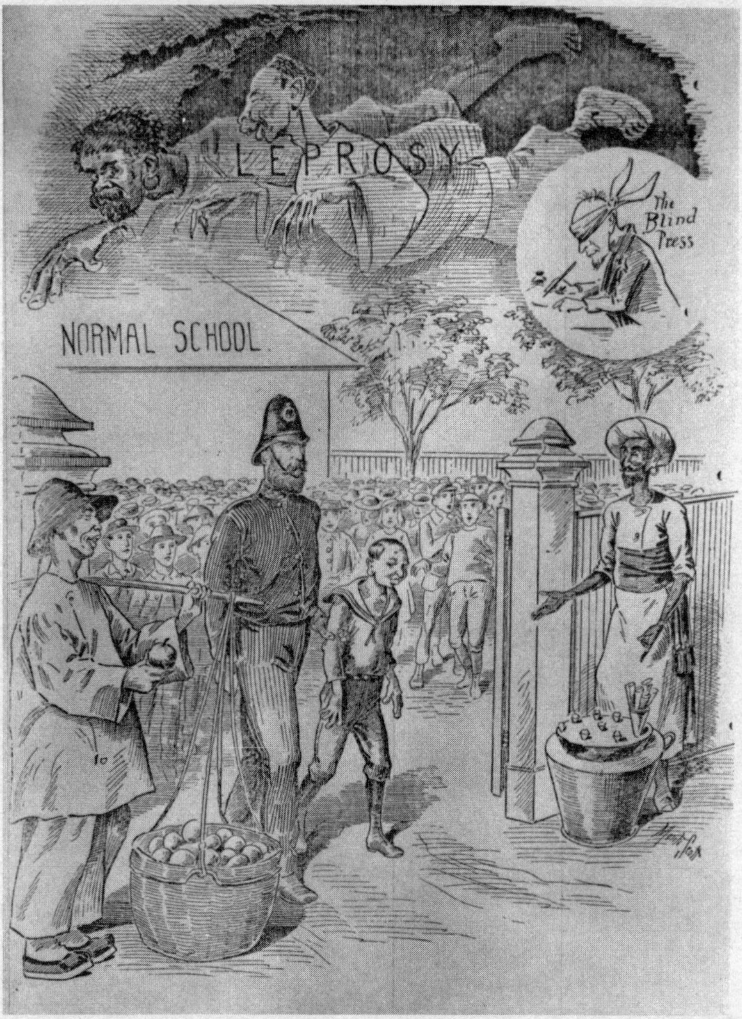

Cartoon from the *Worker* of Christmas 1895 showing how the fear of leprosy aroused racism in Queensland society. The boy leper is snatched from his school. (Courtesy Queensland Parliamentary Library)

> things if a man ran the risk of being committed to a leper station without the greatest precaution being taken to prove that he was suffering from leprosy.

While the leprosy bill was being debated in parliament Eugen Hirschfeld, honorary bacteriologist to the Brisbane Hospital, and Sir Henry Norman, governor of Queensland, shared the forum at a meeting of the Royal Society of Queensland to expound different aspects of the disease. Dr Hirschfeld described the clinical appearance of infection and advocated the establishment of an Australian federal asylum for lepers from all colonies. His Excellency told of his experiences among lepers in India and the West Indies. The *Brisbane Courier* published large extracts of their addresses and added comment of its own in an editorial, part of which read:

> All the evidence proves that in the earlier stages of the disease there is not the slightest cause for alarm, and that the Government may then be especially careful to see that individual life and comfort is not sacrificed to panic. At the same time the very existence of this panic compels a humane Government the more to take under its care the persons of those from whom both friends and hirelings flee. The arrangements now made will secure the comfort of the unfortunate patients; and the last difficulty is removed by the clause providing that the Minister may discharge a person suspected of being a leper on its being proved to his satisfaction that the case is not one of leprosy.

The government then validated its previous actions by proclaiming part of Stradbroke Island and Friday Island as lazarets and formalizing the positions of medical officers, Arthur Salter for Friday Island, and Patrick Smith, superintendent of the Dunwich Benevolent Asylum, for the Stradbroke Island lazaret in the Government Gazette. At first only a few patients were segregated at Stradbroke but their plight according to Smith was an unhappy one for he remarked in a report that "In such a disease, which may be said to be incurable, and which slowly but surely makes progress, many of the patients, as is to be expected, are debilitated and the general health more or less undermined". When leprosy appeared in coloured patients, as it often did, the Queensland public were not greatly perturbed. As the *Worker* put it, "Cases of leprous kanakas and Chinamen, Afghans and coolies may be brought to light every month without occasioning more than a passing comment". However, when an eleven-year-old white boy contracted the disease, more concern was shown. The lad was born on board ship while his parents were migrating to the colony from England. Living all his life in Brisbane, he had attended the Fortitude Valley State School for five years. Shortly after transferring to the Normal School Edward Street in the capital city, he developed signs of the disease. After being confirmed as a case of leprosy he was sent to the Stradbroke Island lazaret where, with five lepers, "he will linger out the remainder of his fearful existence". The *Worker* reported the events in rather sensational words: "The little boy lately taken to Dunwich seems to be affected with the same type of leprosy as the young man Quigley, in whose case the disease is making fearful headway. . . His neck, chest and body are plenteously covered with sores which are calculated to make even a strong stomach revolt. . . Two years ago he was not nearly so bad, and contrasting him with his condition then we should say that it would be kindness to allow him to quietly quit this life which must be a veritable hell." There were to be quite a lot more who contracted the disease and whose lives were most unpleasant, for segregation did not eradicate leprosy as it had done in some countries. Apparently the Queensland climate was very favourable for the growth of the responsible organism and many cases of the infection went undetected and continued to live in the community free to pass on the disease.

In 1907 the government decided to close both lazarets and accommodate all sufferers at Peel Island, one and a half miles to the west of Stradbroke Island, which had previously served as a quarantine station. Shortly after the transfer the inmates numbered eighty-four, of whom twenty were Europeans and the remainder mostly South Sea Islanders and Australian Aborigines. With no known cure for the disease the morale among the patients was very low. A few had natural remissions and were allowed to return to their homes but the majority progressed to a fatal end. Around 1910 there was a change with the news that chaulmoogra oil extracted from a tree which grows in Burma was being used with favourable results in overseas countries. When it was introduced at Peel Island with the same promise spirits rose.

In 1927 the Commonwealth government published a report of an extensive study of leprosy in Australia made by Cecil Cook. Cook was interested in the manner in which the white patients had contracted the disease. At the time of the study it was generally accepted that a second case occurred only after a long period of intimate contact with a leper — generally living with an infected person for weeks, months or even years. Aborigines, convicts, and free settlers from Europe were ruled out by Cook as possible sources of infection. He believed that the natives did not suffer from leprosy until after white man settled in Australia and the absence of leprosy from Europe for centuries made it unlikely that the migrants carried the infection. He then examined the possibility of the disease in Chinese or South Sea Islanders in

Queensland as the origin. He said that the South Sea Islanders kept to themselves and there was seldom any close association with other races in Queensland. Cook postulated that it was a different matter with the Chinese who often persuaded Aboriginal women to live with them in their camps on the goldfields and elsewhere. In this way leprosy was passed on to the Aboriginal women. In the early days of the colony many white men cohabited with Aboriginal women on the fringe of developed areas where women of their own race were scarce. When the native women left the Chinese they spread the disease among their own people and in some instances infected the white men with whom they lived. There is no doubt new cases of leprosy in the white population originated in this way but, as Cook himself admitted, there were several cases where there was no apparent association with lepers either white or coloured. Cook rightly stated that there were many undetected lepers in the community from whom the infection must have been acquired. But even this suggested link was often ruled out. Quigley and the boy leper seemed to have had no long association with any person who could have been even an undetected leper. Later workers have suggested another way that the disease may be spread. It is now believed by such scientists that leprosy may be spread by droplet infection from the nose and throat of a leper as in the case of the common cold. In the case of the common cold, however, few people have any immunity and there are many cases. In leprosy, it is suggested that immunity is quickly developed by most people on exposure and only a very small minority fail to be protected in this way. It is this small minority who develop leprosy without any long association with a leprous person.

Chaulmoogra oil failed to live up to its early promise. After a long trial it was realized that in those cases which seemed to be responding to it the improvement was due to a natural remission. With this realization the attitude among patients returned to one of dejection. In 1940 the government decided to separate the white and coloured lepers. The latter were transferred to Fantome Island near Palm Island north of Townsville. There they were cared for by sisters from the Order of Franciscan Missionaries of Mary. Segregation was still having no effect on the spread of the scourge and by the end of 1944 there were 120 patients in detention of whom 50 were European and 70 coloured. Then came what all had been praying for — an effective drug to treat the disease. Towards the end of the 1940s the use of dapsones, a group of synthetic drugs, was proving successful. By

1950 the total lepers in detention had been reduced from nearly 130 to 46. The new drugs and a change of official attitude towards detention saw Peel Island closed in 1959. Those patients needing isolation or hospital treatment were removed to a ward at Princess Alexandra Hospital, South Brisbane. A few years later those still needing treatment at Fantome Island were found accommodation at the hospital at Palm Island. In 1978 the ward at Princess Alexandra Hospital was no longer needed. A handful of patients needing medical attention went once a week to a clinic at the hospital. Medical science had triumphed over a horrible disease but not before over 700 lepers in Queensland had lived many distressing years in lazarets with the majority of them finally dying a hopeless death.

The First Woman

> The apple of discord is to be cast into our hospitals. A lady — teterrima causa belli — has penetrated to the core of our hospital system, and is determined to effect a permanent lodging. A lady of admirable purpose and highly to be respected for excellent bearing has advanced so far as to have taken courses in Materia Medica and Chemistry at the Middlesex Hospital. . . How should this fair intruder be received? What has already occurred may afford some guide to our conduct. The practical inconveniences, the improprieties, and the anomalies attending the introduction of ladies amongst the classes of male medical students have been so strongly felt, that the students at Middlesex Hospital have revolted against the innovation, and petitioned the lecturers against its continuance. The majority of these gentlemen concurred in the feeling of the students and the further desired privileges have not been accorded.
>
> She is perfectly in earnest, and clearly insensible to the unpleasant feelings which her presence must arouse; for undaunted by her failure at Middlesex Hospital, she has made application at other hospitals. But the same principle is obviously involved wherever the question is to be carried. When all can be said in favour has been heard there will remain the unalterable sense of impropriety in mingling young men with young women in classes destined to see and hear daily sights, descriptions, and explanations which cannot be endured by men in the presence of women, without a violation of all the relations of sex which are essential to the well-being of our social system as at present framed.

With the above words the English medical journal, the *Lancet*, in 1862 expressed its opposition to Elizabeth Garrett, who had the "audacity" to make a determined effort to enter the medical profession. Four years later, when she had overcome the opposition of male students, lecturers, hospitals and at least one examining board to become the first woman to qualify in medicine in England, the *Lancet* begrudgingly saluted "this blue-eyed priestess of Aesculapius". However, it felt sure that "the examiners had due regard for sex, and omitted all those subjects of examination which would be shocking to the female mind, but which are very necessary for ordinary medical practice". The journal also predicted that admission of Miss Garrett as an apothecary would not tempt other young ladies to follow her example.

Opposition to women entering the medical profession was only part of a wider disapproval of the higher education of the fairer sex in the nineteenth century. Those who resisted such attempts were following the example of Queen Victoria who in no uncertain terms expressed the opinion that a woman's place was in the home. Entrance to the professions and in particular to the medical profession was abhorrent to the royal lady. She wrote to her prime minister, Gladstone, advising him that Sir William Jenner, her personal physician, would tell him what an awful idea it was to allow young girls and young men to enter the dissecting room together. But the campaign against the women was unsuccessful and the *Lancet*'s prediction that other young women would not follow Elizabeth Garrett's footsteps proved to be incorrect. Other women demanded entrance to the medical profession and the London School of Medicine for Women was established. The school's association with the Royal Free Hospital provided an easier path for women to enter medicine than England's first woman doctor had trod.

One who followed the new path was Lilian Violet Cooper, daughter of Henry Fallowfield Cooper, a captain in the Royal Marines, and his wife Elizabeth. In 1886, Lilian left her home in Luton, Kent, at the age of twenty-five to live in London to commence her medical course. With her went her close friend, Mary Josephine Bedford, daughter of Captain (later Admiral) George and Eleanor Bedford of Notting Hill, Middlesex. The two shared lodgings in Russell Square and while Lilian Cooper went to her lectures in medicine Josephine Bedford studied painting. When Lilian Cooper completed her medical course in 1890, the English colleges of physicians and of surgeons were still refusing women permission to sit for their conjoint diploma in medicine and surgery. Women were forced to journey to Scotland or Ireland where the colleges were more favourably disposed to the idea of female doctors. Lilian Cooper chose Scotland and after passing the conjoint examinations of the Royal College of Physicians and of the Royal College of Surgeons, Edinburgh, and the faculty of Physicians and Surgeons, Glasgow, she received a licentiate from Edinburgh. She was now Dr Lilian Cooper.

Her first position after qualifying was as an assistant to a general practitioner at Halstead, Essex. She soon found that she was to make up to thirty home visits on foot each day. All the night calls fell to her lot and often involved a trudge of two or three miles over snow-covered, ploughed fields. After a few months of this unsatisfactory position she went to London to consult the dean of her medical school who, after marriage, was now Mrs Elizabeth Garrett Anderson. Dr Anderson had just received a letter from James Booth, a general medical practitioner in South Brisbane, Queensland, asking her to select a woman doctor as an assistant. After a visit to Australia in 1885, Dr Anderson was conversant with medical practice in the colonies and suggested to the young woman doctor that she consider migrating to take the position. Dr Booth had also written to Lady Musgrave, wife of Sir Anthony Musgrave who had returned to England in 1888 after serving as governor of Queensland for five years. Dr Cooper favoured the idea and was interviewed by Lady Musgrave who with Dr Anderson believed that Miss Cooper would measure up to what had been requested — a really good and competent medical woman. She accepted the offer and Josephine Bedford decided to go with her to Queensland. The *Halstead and Colne Valley Gazette* of 26 February 1891 expressed regret at the loss the town would sustain and referred to her in warm terms. When she left many of the people assembled to see her off and wish her bon voyage. The two ladies left Plymouth on 10 April 1891 in the Orient Line's RMS *Lusitania* under the command of Captain H.E. Inskip. (It was not the Cunard Line *Lusitania* which was sunk in World War I.) Sailing through the Suez Canal the vessel arrived in Sydney on 25 May. Transferring to the AUSN steamer *Aramac*, Dr Cooper and her companion arrived in Brisbane four days later. The first step was to present her certificates to the Queensland Medical Board with an application for registration. At its meeting on 4 June 1891, the board approved her application and she became the first woman doctor in Queensland.

Unfortunately, once again the position proved unsatisfactory. The main difficulty, — rumour had it — was her employer's addiction to alcohol. Again she had the courage to do something about it. She had the contract dissolved. But, what should she do next? The Brisbane medical profession boycotted her, not because she had left the position but because she was a woman. There was only one action to take — to set up practice on her own. Under the circumstances it was a brave decision. But she went ahead and on Christmas Eve 1891, the readers of the *Brisbane Courier* noted in the morning's issue the following advertisement:

Dr Lilian Cooper, L.R.C.P. and L.R.C.S., Edin., L.F.P. and S. Glasg.,

> having resigned her assistantship to Dr Booth, has COMMENCED PRACTICE in Brisbane. Consulting Rooms, 5 George St., Mansions. Hours, 11 a.m. to 3 p.m. Private Residence Russell St. South Brisbane, Hours 8.30 a.m. to 10 a.m. and 6 to 8 p.m. Dr Cooper has made a special study of the Diseases of Women and Children.

Progress in the new practice was slow. She was soon aware that those prejudices against women doctors that had accompanied their entry into the profession in England also existed in Brisbane. The professional boycott continued for two years. When she attempted to join the Queensland Medical Society, the precursor of the Queensland branch of the British Medical Association, her application was rejected. At last, at the general meeting of the society on 13 June 1893, she attended as a visitor. Despite the fact that the rules stated that any qualified medical practitioner resident in Queensland was eligible for election as a member, a spirited debate resulted when Dr Cooper's name was submitted. Finally Dr (later Sir) David Hardie proposed her admission and his motion was accepted and carried. The initial attitude of the Queensland Medical Society is not surprising when it is compared with that prevailing in England at the time. It was only a year before Dr Cooper's acceptance by the professional body in Brisbane that the British Medical Association in England had expunged from the articles of the association the clause that read, "No female shall be eligible for election as a member of the Association". Most of the Brisbane public were also slow to accept the idea of a woman doctor. But the trickle of patients who did overcome prejudice and attend the new doctor found that behind a mannish figure and brusque manner there was a kind and competent practitioner. They found also that they could rely on Dr Cooper to visit no matter what hour of the day or night she was called and no matter what distance she had to travel. In those years she used all manner of transport to reach her patients. The striding figure of the tall woman doctor with her Assam silk dust-coat flying in the breeze gradually became a familiar sight as she visited the homes of patients near her practice. Visits to more distant suburbs were made by horse and sulky. At night she risked her neck by riding a bicycle. An elderly resident of Mount Mee related how Dr Cooper rode over thirty miles sidesaddle to attend her as a child. Then with the introduction of the motor car in the early years of the twentieth century, she joined many male doctors who pioneered with their five and seven horsepower Oldsmobiles, their eight horsepower Glides, their De Dions,

Darracqs and Ramblers. Dr Cooper drove an Oldsmobile and when it broke down as often happened in the early days of motoring, she is said to have used language unbecoming a lady.

Lilian Cooper was the only woman doctor in Queensland for ten years. In May 1901 she was joined by Eleanor Greenham, and the two were at first also Brisbane's only women drivers. Dr Greenham was the first of twenty-two women out of a total of four hundred and thirty-five doctors to be registered in the state in the first decade of the twentieth century. Some of them were quite venturesome, taking up practice in remote areas. In 1906 Mabel Crutchfield went to Boulia and Mary Edelstan to Jundah. The next year Laura Weir commenced practising at Springsure and Mary de Garis at Muttaburra. They were followed by Ada Griffiths who hung up her plate at Adavale in 1908. By this time Lilian Cooper was well established and many wives of prominent men in Brisbane and country squatters either attended her themselves or took their children for advice.

Dr Cooper's interest in women and children was manifest in her appointments to hospitals, the first being to the Hospital for Sick Children. Through the efforts of Mary McConnell, it had been opened in 1878 in a rented building in Leichhardt Street Brisbane, later the site of the Presbyterian Church. By the time Dr Cooper arrived in Brisbane, the hospital had been transferred to Herston, where in 1883 a new building was erected for its purpose. The 1896 annual report of the hospital committee, composed solely of women, stated that "it was found necessary to ask for additional assistance in the Outpatient Department and the appointment of Dr Lilian Cooper gave general satisfaction". Dr Cooper served as an honorary medical officer for twenty years after which she was retained as a consultant surgeon. Once, when there was a shortage of staff, she resided at the hospital and combined the duties of resident medical officer with her private practice. On 1 November 1900, Lilian Cooper and her colleague David Hardie, who had proposed her membership of the Queensland Medical Society, were present at the opening of a new hospital to be devoted solely to the diseases of women. The two doctors were the hospital's first honorary officers. It was to be conducted temporarily in two cottages in Leichhardt Street not far from the building which had served as the first children's hospital. Lady Lamington, the wife of the governor of Queensland at the time, had given the project her blessing and she was to be honoured in its name. Later the first honoraries were to be joined by Joseph Bancroft and Wilton Love and when the committee gave Dr

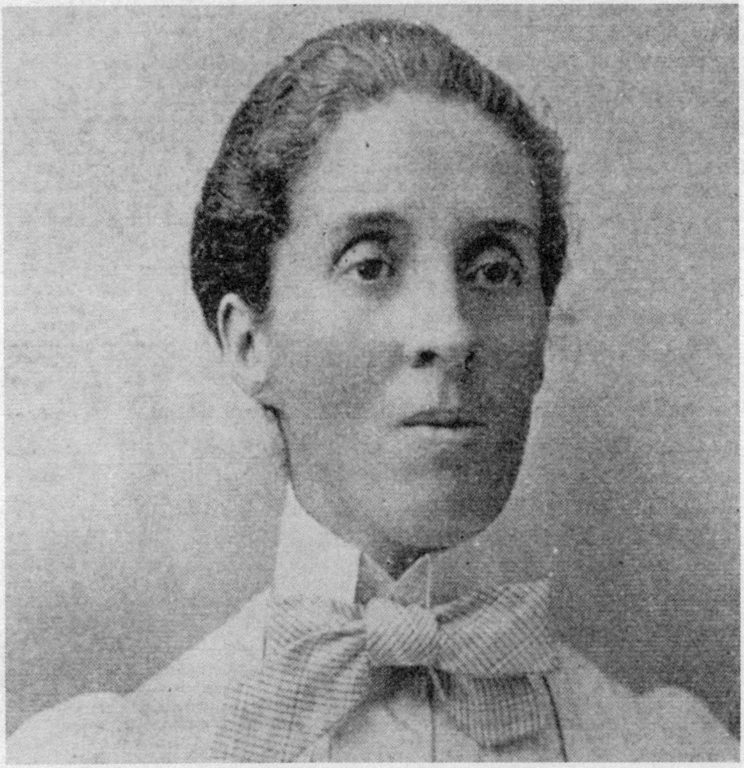

Queensland's first woman doctor, Dr Lilian Cooper. From Queensland Biographical Sketches 1900. (Courtesy Oxley Library)

Cooper leave to go overseas in 1904 she was relieved by William Byrne, the chairman of the obstetrics and gynaecology section of the British Medical Association in Queensland. When Lilian Cooper returned to the staff of the Lady Lamington Hospital twelve months later it was functioning in new quarters specially built for it in St Paul's Terrace. Dr Cooper gave excellent service to these two hospitals but the hospital with which she was most closely associated was the Mater Misericordiae. When the Sisters of Mercy established their hospital in a double-storeyed building on North Quay, called at first Aubigney and later Loretto in 1906, Dr Cooper did not initially send any patients there. She attended the hospital only when one of her patients insisted that she would be nursed nowhere else. From that beginning Lilian Cooper became the greatest benefactor among the doctors that the Mater Hospital had in its early years. She sent all her patients there and when the Sisters of Mercy crossed the river to establish their hospital on Mater Hill, South Brisbane, Lilian Cooper followed, one of her patients being among the first to be admitted when the Mater Private Hospital was opened in 1910. She became a member of the Mater Hospital medical board and a senior honorary surgeon. While Dr Cooper always retained her interest in diseases of women and children, she gradually also developed a great skill as a surgeon — an unusual specialty for a woman.

In 1906 Lilian Cooper purchased a two-storeyed residence, Auckland House, at the corner of George and Mary streets. Here she lived and practised for twenty years. It was here, too, that her lifelong companion, Miss Bedford, formed a base for her charity work. The first meeting of the Queensland National Council of Women was held at Auckland House soon after the two women took residence there. Ten years before, Miss Bedford had been elected to the committee of the Hospital for Sick Children, on which she served for twenty-five years, becoming a vice-president in 1920. The organization with which Josephine Bedford was most closely associated was the Playground and Recreation Association. At a meeting of the National Council of Women in 1913 a provisional committee to found the playground association was appointed with Miss Bedford as convenor. The first playground was opened at Paddington in 1918 and three years later a second was opened at Spring Hill.

Apart from her 1904 trip Dr Cooper made two other visits overseas. Accompanied by Miss Bedford she travelled to England in 1911 via the United States of America. While the doctor visited the Mayo Clinic in Minnesota and the John Hopkins Hospital in Maryland her companion studied the playground movement, attending a summer school in San Francisco. In England, Lilian Cooper was awarded a doctorate of medicine at the Durham University. The two women were back in Brisbane two years when World War I broke out. They went to the United Kingdom again in 1915 and both joined the Scottish Women's Hospital and were posted to Macedonia. There the doctor worked as a surgeon in an allied hospital and Miss Bedford drove an ambulance. The King of Serbia recognized their services by awarding them the Order of St Sava.

Returning to Brisbane the two women resumed their former life, the doctor resuming her medical practice and her companion her charitable work. In 1918 Dr Cooper operated on a woman for appendicitis. Four years later the patient's husband wrote to the doctor, claiming that a Newcastle surgeon, William Nickson, had removed a pair of surgical forceps from his wife's abdomen, and alleging that Dr Cooper had left them there after the appendicectomy. Dr Cooper ignored the letter. A few weeks later the man appeared in the surgeon's rooms demanding compensation. Lilian Cooper characteristically said, "You'll have to prove it". She was sued for negligence and £2,500 compensation was claimed. The case came before Mr Justice Lukin and a jury of four in the Brisbane Supreme Court on 29 May 1923. The patient was represented by Mr H.D. Macrossan while Dr Cooper was defended by Mr Feez KC. The patient submitted that she had suffered recurrent pain since Dr Cooper had removed her appendix which was the only operation she had undergone until the one in which the forceps were removed. Dr Nickson confirmed that on 5 August 1922 he had removed a pair of forceps with the handle of one flange missing from the plaintiff's abdomen. In his opening address, Dr Cooper's counsel pointed out that she was a surgeon of great experience who had performed over one thousand abdominal operations. A number of these had taken place during the recent war, during the time that his client was a senior surgeon at an army hospital near Salonika. Two prominent members of Brisbane's medical profession, Donald Cameron and Edwin Ahearn, testified that although a surgeon accepted overall responsibility during an operation, it was the duty of the theatre sister to check the instruments before the abdomen was closed. Both doctors commented on Dr Cooper's ability as a surgeon, Dr Ahearn stating that she possessed competency and skill of a high order. Sister Mary Augustine, theatre sister for thirteen years at the Mater Hospital before 1918, testified that she had found all instruments correct at the end of the appendix operation and that the forceps exhibited in court were stamped Zoeller and Co. and no forceps of this brand were used in the Mater Hospital theatre. The latter evidence was confirmed by Sister Mary Lucienne, matron of the hospital. After several retirements, the jury found that there was no negligence on the part of Dr Cooper or any other person. Some years later, Sir Clarence Leggett, an eminent Brisbane surgeon, was examining a woman at the Brisbane Princess Alexandra Hospital. Noticing the operation scars on her abdomen, he commented, "You have been in the wars," whereupon the patient opened her locker and produced a pair of battered forceps. Waving them at Sir Clarence, she said, "This is why. Dr Cooper left these inside me, when she operated on me for appendicitis".

The case did not affect Dr Cooper's reputation, but the next year, aged sixty-three, she retired from the Mater Hospital consultant staff. In 1927, her skill as a surgeon was recognized by her admission as foundation fellow of the Royal Australasian College of Surgeons — an honour that only a small number of women hold. In the same year the residence in George Street was sold and later it became the temporary headquarters of the tuberculosis division of the state health department. The two women purchased Old St Mary's in Main Street, Kangaroo Point adjoining the lovely stone Anglican Church of St Mary, the Virgin. Old St Mary's was built by the Reverend Robert Moffatt, Rector of the first Anglican Church in John Street, Kangaroo Point. When the new St Mary's Church was built in 1873, a new rectory was established closer to it than the Reverend Moffatt's original home. The two friends lived in their new residence in semi-retirement, Lilian Cooper seeing a few patients and Josephine Bedford pursuing her voluntary work with less vigour. After retiring completely in 1941, Queensland's first woman doctor died at home on 18 August 1947 at the age of eight-six. She was buried in the Toowong cemetery with Anglican rites. Miss Bedford was now the sole owner of Old St Mary's. She attended the services at St Mary's Church regularly and honoured her life-long friend through gifts to the Warrior Chapel there. Dr Cooper's medal which she was awarded by the King of Serbia is displayed on the altar frontal. But Miss Bedford had more ambitious plans to honour Dr Cooper. Before the doctor's death, they had often discussed what would become of their property when they had both gone. They had agreed that it should be used for the care of the aged and the sick. An organization was needed to carry out their wishes. There may have been some tentative discussions with their own Anglican church but there is no record of these having gone past the conversation stage. Dr Cooper had often discussed the idea with the Mater Hospital Sisters but they were committed with the needs to expand their own hospital with plans for the Children's and the Mater Mothers' hospitals. Miss Bedford discussed the subject with the Sisters of Charity who had already purchased land at Enoggera for a hospice for the age and dying. That land was sold and the Mount Olivet hospital was established by the order on the site of Old St Mary's. Miss Bedford was present at the laying of the foundation stone on 24 October 1954, but she did not live to see the hospital completed, dying at the age of ninety-four on 22 December 1955. When the hospital was opened in 1957, a second site where Dr Cooper had lived was used for medical purposes. A reminder of this is seen in the inscription on the plaque opposite the foundation stone.

THE LAND ON WHICH
THIS HOSPITAL WAS BUILT
WAS GIVEN AS A MEMORIAL TO
THE LIFE AND WORK OF
LILIAN V. COOPER, M.D., F.R.A.C.S.
BY HER FRIEND
M.J. BEDFORD

The two women are also honoured in the Marycrest Retirement Centre which the Sisters of Charity opened next to Mount Olivet in 1977. An activities centre on the ground floor is named in honour of Miss Bedford and on the top floor is the Lilian Cooper Nursing Home. Josephine Bedford loved trees, and the Women's Historical Society, of which she was a keen member, remembered this when they planted a bottle tree in her honour in the grounds of Newstead House. The inscription on a marker nearby reads:

THIS TREE
was planted on 22 March 1966 by
LADY LAVARACK
Wife of Queensland's first Brisbane-born Governor
and first Patroness of the Women's Historical Association
As a memorial to
MISS MARY JOSEPHINE BEDFORD
Honorary life member
Who died on 22 December 1955.
A sylvan scene and, as the ranks assume
Shade above shade a woody theatre of stateliest view.
Milton, Paradise Lost

Black Death

Samuel Pepys, the English diarist, wrote in his journal on 7 June 1665:

> This day, much against my will, I did in Drury Lane see two or three houses marked with a red cross upon the doors and "Lord have mercy upon us" writ there; which was a sad sight to me, being the first of the kind that to my remembrance, I ever saw. It put me into an ill conception of myself and my smell, so that I was forced to buy some roll-tobacco to smell and chaw, which took away the apprehension.

It was the year of the Great Plague of London and Pepys was describing one of the measures taken to combat the pestilence. The true nature of infectious disease was then unknown. It was believed that it was God's vengeance on a sinful people. But the people knew that the disease was passed on in some way from those suffering from it. When a case of plague was diagnosed, not only was a red cross painted on the door and a prayer written, but the whole household was locked inside and a guard was posted outside to ensure no member escaped. It was generally a certain method of assuring that all in the house died. Another belief at the time was that domestic animals were in some way the cause of the scourge and two pence were paid for every dog and cat caught and killed. Meanwhile, the millions of rats that infested the city — the true source of the disease — were unmolested and the disease was passed on from infected rats to human patients by the bites of fleas. At times a death occurred before any diagnosis was made and a message was taken to the sexton for a grave to be dug and the bells tolled for a burial. It was the sexton's duty in such cases to send searchers to the house to determine the cause. They were usually old women, who worked in pairs and carried white staffs as badges of office. Their presence in the street warned the neighbours of possible danger. As the number of cases grew all those who could manage fled the city. King Charles II first went to Hampton Court. When signs of the disease appeared close he transferred to Salisbury and later to Oxford. Only one minister stayed in London to carry out the affairs of state. Others who remained in the city were the drivers of the plague carts and their cries of "bring out your dead" were heard as the carts rumbled through the streets at night. The doors of the afflicted houses were opened and a coffin was pushed out into the street. Sometimes the body was covered in a shroud. Often there was no covering at all.

The exact number who died from the scourge is not known. There were many possibilities for error. Some estimates reached 100,000 from a population of 350,000. The weekly totals increased as the summer continued. At the end of August, Pepys wrote:

> Thus this month ends with great sadness upon the publick, through the greatness of the plague everywhere throughout the kingdom almost. Every day sadder and sadder news of the increase. In the city this week, 7496 and of them 6102 of the plague.

With the arrival of the cooler months of the winter of 1665–66 the incidence of the disease lessened and finally the epidemic was over. Plague then disappeared altogether from London. Some authorities believe that the Great Fire of London that occurred the next year was responsible, killing all the rats that harboured the plague germs. Others suggest that the reason for the disappearance was the arrival of the fierce grey rat which drove out the black rat which was the source of plague.

When Governor Phillip brought the First Fleet of convicts to New South Wales in 1788 his unwilling immigrants brought with them many of the diseases from which they had suffered in the British Isles. Many of the willing immigrants who followed later also helped in the transfer. They brought tuberculosis, typhoid fever and the childhood diseases but not plague, for it had not reappeared in their native land. For over a century after the arrival of Governor Phillip and the first batch of convicts, plague did not cross the shores of Australia. However, in 1893, a plague epidemic began in Hong Kong and over the next few years it spread to many countries bounding the Pacific Ocean. It came to Australia in 1900 carried by rats on ships from one or more of the places where the scourge was raging to infect the Australian rats and then to be passed on to the human population. In January suspected cases of the disease in humans were reported in Adelaide and Sydney. The case in Adelaide was not confirmed but the Sydney patient was definitely suffering from plague.

No human case occurred in Brisbane for another three months. During those months the threat of an epidemic was discussed in many quarters. The Central Board of Health which included in its membership prominent Brisbane medical practitioners decided that two of its members, John Thomson and Wilton Love, should prepare a pamphlet couched in simple terms to inform the public of the true nature of the disease. By 1900, the medical profession was in a position to tell the Queensland community that the germ that caused plague had been identified and that in an epidemic it first infected rats and was transferred to humans by the bites of fleas. To prevent its occurrence every step must be taken to destroy the rat population — no rats, no plague. Besides preparing pamphlets, the Central Board of Health issued recommendations and promulgated regulations. But it did not have the power to enforce them. Members attended meetings of the board in a part-time capacity and there was no state health department employing experts in public health. It was expected that local authorities or joint epidemic boards consisting of representatives of a number of neighbouring councils would carry out the recommendations and police the regulations.

The enthusiasm with which this was done varied considerably. This was a reflection of the attitude towards health adopted by the various governments in the developing colony. The early legislators were concerned with distributing the land, building railways, regulating goldfields and developing an education system. Health had a low priority. In the 1860s when a health bill was introduced into parliament, Herbert, the colonial secretary, arranged for it to lapse as he considered there was no need for such legislation. A smallpox scare in 1872 was necessary to frighten the government into passing the first Health Act which proved to be almost useless. It was in force only after special promulgation and then only for six months unless the promulgation was repeated. The Brisbane Municipal Council, after being forced to have the act promulgated in its area, finally persuaded the government not to renew its application. This neglect and lack of interest in health provided such a favourable medium for the development of filth diseases that typhoid fever raged for a number of years. Its incidence again frightened the government into action and another health act was passed in 1884. The new legislation was an improvement on the first attempt but it still had the weakness of not providing for a central executive to see that its provisions were enforced.

After the report of definite cases of plague in Sydney, the Queensland press gave almost daily reports of the progress of the disease there and published several editorials giving its views of

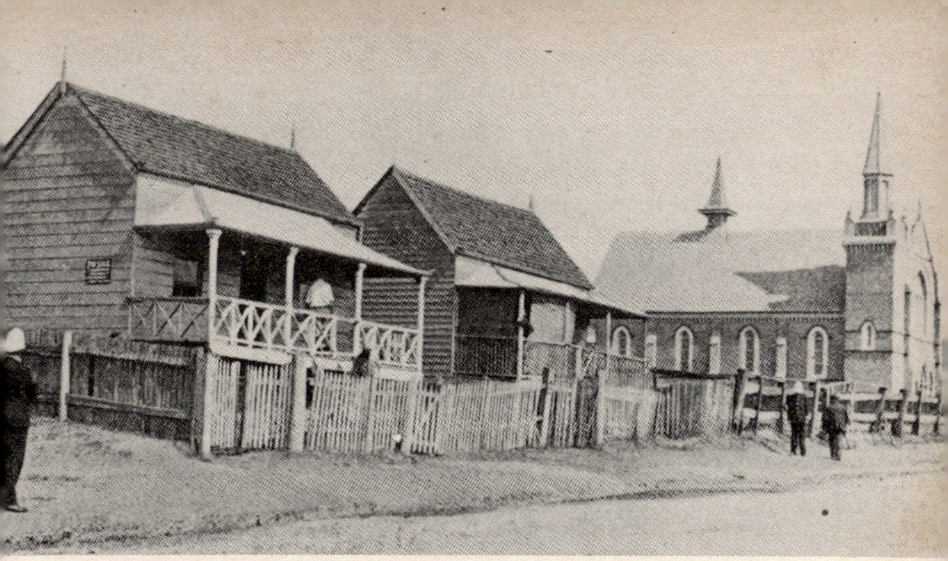

This photograph showed readers of the *Queenslander* that the plague could strike any home. Brisbane's first plague victim lived in the house on the left in Woolloongabba in 1900. (Courtesy Oxley Library)

what should done in Queensland. The *Brisbane Courier* editorial followed a meeting of the Central Board of Health:

> The truth, however, is that the seriousness of the situation lies, as it always does, not in the actual presence of the disease, but in the presence of the conditions which give it a foothold and encouragement. . .
>
> The point calling for attention is the manner in which people ignorant or careless of sanitation live among ourselves. The greatest danger lies with those who from their racial habits or cheapness, huddle together in filth. The low-class Chinaman, the Indian or Syrian hawker, in less degree the walk-about Kanaka want our first attention.

Health authorities barricaded the Woolloongabba home of the first plague victim. From the *Queenslander* of 1900. (Courtesy Oxley Library)

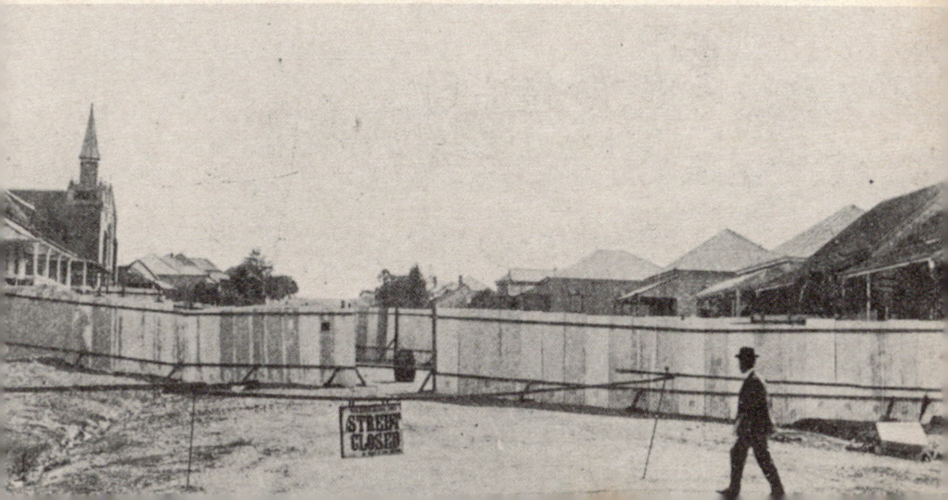

> The hovels in which these men congregate should be raided in the interest of cleanliness and health. Next to these come certain other houses as far from godliness as cleanliness. Then there are a number of low-class white lodging houses which want close inspection. Dr Thomson and others at Wednesday's meeting spoke of the filthy state of the backyards in Queen Street itself. There ought to be a universal inspection of backyards.

The *Brisbane Courier* correctly associated plague with filth, but it omitted to state that it was a special kind of filth which favoured the development of the disease. It was the filth that provided breeding places for rats. The Queensland country press echoed the rather racist editorial of the Brisbane paper. The *Townsville Bulletin* said:

> In north Queensland ports, where the disease may now any day appear, it is assuredly incumbent on the local authorities to carefully watch those neighbourhoods where Asiatics and Polynesians congregate. We stand in greater danger from the bubonic plague here than do other portions of Australia, because of the larger proportion of these races in our population. A comparatively small expenditure now will be the best safeguard against the very heavy expenditure that the appearance of the plague among the coloured people would necessitate.

The *Mackay Chronicle* was also certain that the danger lay among the coloured people whom white man had so eagerly brought to Queensland to work on the sugar plantations:

> Provision must be made to localise the Kanakas in our midst by retaining them on the plantations where they work and forbidding movement therefrom without passes duly signed. Furthermore, strict rules in regard to bathing on the part of Polynesians should be enforced, and it is hoped that as soon as possible action in this and other directions urgently required will be taken.

In subsequent editorials the *Brisbane Courier* corrected its omission of the relationship of rats to plague and on 27 February reported that the suggestion of the Central Board of Health that all rats should be destroyed was being followed by the Brisbane and South Brisbane municipal councils as well as the Booroodabin divisional board. A crusade against the rodents had been started by the authorities especially in the vicinity of wharves. In addition the Brisbane council raised the bounty paid to individuals for dead rats from two pence to sixpence.

The reaction of Queensland citizens to the threat, and later the occurrence of plague, may be gauged from accounts written at or near the time. Burnett Ham, the first Queensland health commissioner wrote in 1907 that "the outbreak of plague in Brisbane in 1900, and the scare, alarm and excitement of the populace, even at a name whose association conjures up fearful visions of the *Black Death* of the middle ages, led to an urgent demand for sanitary reform". This statement suggests that the people were in a state of great panic. But Ham did not come to Brisbane until the next year and from other accounts it appears that he exaggerated the position. There is no doubt that some Queenslanders had read of the pestilence that devastated Europe in the fourteenth century. Some may even have read Daniel Defoe's picturesque *Journal of the Plague Year* or Samuel Pepys's more exact description in his diary. But Ham himself said that when the people were offered protection through inoculation the indifference shown led to its abandonment. The *Brisbane Courier* believed the people were more interested in the Boer War, and in the Queensland volunteers joining the British in South Africa.

> It is a matter for thankfulness that the visitation had come with the war. Had there been nothing to distract our thoughts this particular trouble might breed a panic; and instead of taking the plague quietly, and in common-sense fashion, the community would have been working up to such a pitch that the thing we dread would have had an easy entrance. Nothing is more certain than that fear is the handmaid of death. When people can look disease fairly in the face they often disarm it, and at the present juncture we are half-way to victory by being calm and dispassionately taking stock of the situation.

One wonders whether the people were distracted by the *Courier*'s reports of "gallant little Mafeking besieged by the Boers"; of the retreating Boer columns under Commandant De Wit and Botha after their defeat near Wepener with the English in hot pursuit; and of the report that the British commander-in-chief, Lord Roberts, held a position of supreme advantage. Perhaps the reason for the absence of panic was the fact that Queenslanders had become used to epidemic diseases. In the 1890s over six hundred were dying in the colony each year from tuberculosis in its various forms. Typhoid fever and diphtheria had claimed hundreds each year and each year one baby in ten died before reaching one year of age. They had been told that the medical profession knew much more about plague than in days gone past. When the first case occurred in Brisbane, the citizens did not avoid the afflicted house as their ancestors had done when the plague was raging in England. The *Brisbane Courier* made a report of what happened when the first patient from Woolloongabba was diagnosed: "Notwithstanding the horror which people have of plague, the scene was visited by large numbers of people during Saturday whose curiosity had caused to collect a little distance off and gaze with a peculiar interest at the spot, where the plague fiend has chosen to make his presence felt."

The priority which the governments had given to the health of the citizens of Queensland is exemplified in the appointment of Charles Pound, the first government bacteriologist. When he took up duty in 1893, his duties were to carry out research into the diseases of animals, not humans. The government believed that the health of cattle, horses, sheep and pigs was more important in the development of the colony than the health of its citizens. However, the medical profession convinced the government that Pound should pay attention to human disease and he was doing this by 1900 when plague broke out. The first cases in Sydney prompted the Central Board of Health to ask Pound to examine the rats of Brisbane for evidence of plague. Early in March he made the unwelcome discovery of plague in a black rat found dead in a shop close to a wharf where vessels from Sydney had recently arrived. This finding was an indication that cases would soon occur in the human population. The first patient from Woolloongabba was a van driver employed in removing goods from the same wharf where the dead rat was found.

The Brisbane patient was not the first to contract the disease in Queensland. On 17 April 1900, the head steward on the steamer *Burweh*, a coastal vessel carrying passengers from Sydney to Rockhampton calling en route at Brisbane, was diagnosed as suffering from plague when the vessel reached its destination. On removing the lining of the steward's cabin several dead rats were found. This first case was followed by thirty-five more in Rockhampton before the end of the year. Not long afterwards a steward on another ship, the *Cintra*, also showed certain signs of the disease when the vessel berthed in Townsville. He was the first of thirty-seven cases to occur in that city. Jefferis Turner, an eminent Brisbane doctor, volunteered to go north to act as bacteriologist and confirmed many of the cases by microscopic examination. The Townsville city fathers found that Turner's sobriquet of Gentle Annie was a misnomer when the apparently gentle doctor gave them a piece of his mind when after three weeks they had taken no action on his recommendation to clean the city and destroy all rats. In each of the three centres,

Brisbane, Rockhampton and Townsville, the first cases were in patients who in some way were connected with the wharves. Then cases occurred in Spring Hill, Wickham Terrace, Red Hill and Paddington. The extension into these areas was explained in an interesting report from Arthur Halford, medical officer to the Metropolitan Joint Epidemic Board.

> There is an old sewer which was once an open one, built of brick many years ago, and more recently converted into a covered drain, which collects the drainage from a considerable area of Spring Hill and Wickham Terrace. There are many imperfections in this sewer, and a number of untrapped connections. It empties into the Brisbane River under Collin's Wharf at Petrie's Bight. Cases of plague have occurred along the course of this sewer, and, though chronological order does not show it, there is a complete chain of cases commencing in the neighbourhood of the wharf and the embouchure of the sewer, and including those along its course to the district in which the drain commences. It is likely, however, the communities of rats along the course of the sewer were infected from the wharf rats entering this highway, and from the resulting local infusion, cases among human beings occurred in the neighbourhood. On the Milton side of Brisbane, leading from the lower part of Petrie Terrace to the river, near Boundary Street, is a very old and defective sewer. Cases have occurred on the river road near where this sewer discharges, and there is a continuous chain of cases through Petrie Terrace to the farthermost part of Red Hill and parts of Paddington. In this way the extension along these defective sewers have accounted for the concentration of cases in Spring Hill and Petrie Terrace.

When the epidemic threatened, the joint epidemic board build a plague hospital at Colmslie. When the patients arrived they were attended by doctors and nurses suitably inoculated whilst their contacts were isolated in tents in the grounds. Police were posted to keep intruders out and contacts in. Shortly after the first patient's removal from his home in Woolloongabba, officers from the joint board arrived to cleanse and fumigate the house thoroughly. The whole of the bedding, linen and bed curtains were removed and burnt to ashes in the yard. A barricade of galvanized iron was erected around the victim's and nearby dwellings. Shortly after this was completed, a clergyman from the country, not understanding the purpose of the barricade, stepped through a gap with the intention of taking a short-cut, only to find himself immediately detained by a policeman on guard within the enclosure. Eventually, the cleric was allowed his liberty on his promising to thoroughly disinfect himself and report next morning for medical examination.

The next day, a neatly dressed woman with a baby in her arms saw a horse-drawn bus with people aboard stop in Ann Street, Brisbane. Believing it to be her usual way of travelling home, she climbed aboard. A mounted trooper rode up behind and the bus moved on. She learnt with great concern she had joined a group of contacts being taken to the Colmslie hospital for quarantine. When the bus stopped at the next corner, she alighted but the trooper detained her, unsure of what he should do. He faced a dilemma. He needed advice but he could not leave his post. In a few minutes, a newspaper reporter appeared on a bicycle. At the trooper's request he set off for the police headquarters to report the situation. The sergeant in charge could not act without the orders of the commissioner, to whose house a constable was sent. Meanwhile, back at the bus, the young woman had burst into tears and the baby was crying its head off. After an hour a message came from the commissioner, who had phoned Dr Bancroft, that the poor woman should be allowed to go. The *Brisbane Courier*, reporting the incident, suggested that the bus should be painted yellow to prevent a recurrence of what had happened.

Unidentifiable behind their protective masks, the public health commissioner, Dr Burnett Ham, and his staff prepare to investigate an outbreak of plague in 1905. (Courtesy Queensland Department of Health)

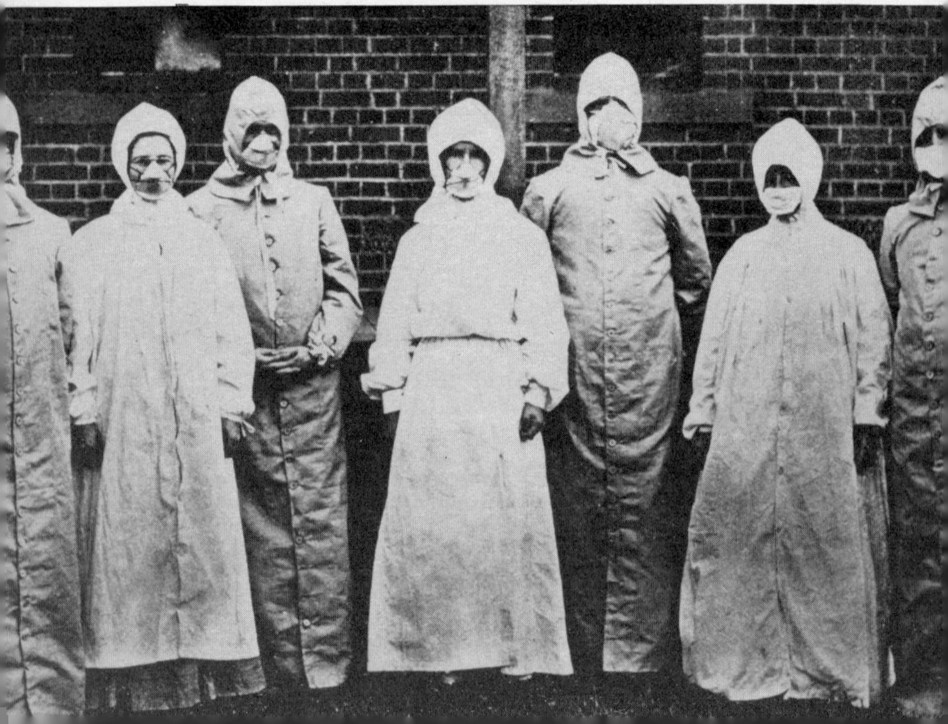

And so the first case of plague in Brisbane was handled with great zeal by doctors from the Central Board of Health, the mayor as chairman of the joint epidemic board and the police. The press reported every aspect of the Brisbane cases as well as giving accounts from Townsville and Rockhampton where other cases had occurred and from Cairns where it was expected the disease had appeared. However, events over the next few days indicated that the administration was not as efficient as it first seemed. When a second case occurred on the following Sunday there was no one available to deal with the patient and he was sent home. The mayor, who really held the reins of power from his position on the epidemic board, was at Sandgate recuperating from the effects of inoculation against the disease. Wilton Love, medical secretary of the central health board was likewise indisposed. As a result, there was no one available to order the patient's transfer to the Colmslie Plague Hospital. Then a coastal vessel, the *Maranoa*, tied up at a Brisbane wharf and disembarked passengers. One of them walked to Dr Bancroft's surgery and was diagnosed as suffering from plague. Next day, there was a search for all who had left the ship. Those who could be found were quarantined at the plague hospital. J.S. (Boss) Badger, manager of the tramways, sought advice on how to disinfect his trams and depot. After a fruitless search, he went ahead himself. It was this indecision that prompted a number of citizens to urge the mayor to call a mass meeting of the inhabitants of Brisbane to solve the lack of leadership. The readers of the *Brisbane Courier* of 3 May were advised in the following manner:

> MASS MEETING OF CITIZENS
> FOR FORMATION OF VIGILANCE COMMITTEE
> CHAIRMAN:- HIS WORSHIP THE MAYOR
>
> Speakers:- Hons. E.B. Forrest and T. Macdonald-Paterson, Members for the City; The Mayor of South Brisbane; John Leahy, Esq., M.L.A.; President Chamber of Commerce: Dr E.S. Jackson, M.B., B.S.: Edwyn Lilley, Esq.; Barrister-At-Law: Rev. T. Nesbit; and J.S. Stoddart Esq., M.L.A., Chairman Brisbane Hospital.
>
> PREVENTION of BUBONIC PLAGUE

The small attendance at the meeting was another indication that the citizens of Brisbane were not unduly alarmed by the threat of the epidemic. However, those who attended listened to prominent men voice dissatisfaction at the way the problem had been tackled and suggest the remedy needed. John Leahy, president of the Chamber of Commerce, considered that there was too much overlapping. Consequently, anything like agreement was out of the question. He praised the work of the mayor, who incidentally was chairing the meeting, but doubted the usefulness of the Central Board of Health and the Joint Epidemic Board. Leahy also questioned whether Justin Foxton, the home secretary and therefore in charge of health matters, had rendered any more service than those two bodies. They were all remarkable for their differences of opinion with no power to enforce their opinions. Sandford Jackson, medical superintendent of the Brisbane Hospital, told the meeting that what was needed was a central authority — an expert health authority — which should give directions. The authority should be in one man.

A vigilance committee was formed and in the next three months joined with the central health board and the municipal council in urging the government to amend the Health Act to establish the central authority recommended by Sandford Jackson. In this advocacy firm support came from the *Brisbane Courier* at frequent intervals. In August 1900, the government heeded the cries and amended the legislation. As a result Bertie Burnett Ham, an expert in sanitary science, came from England to take up duty as Queensland's first public health commissioner. Ham immediately began a vigorous campaign to cope with the disease. When he found local authorities were slow in implementing the plague regulations that he promulgated he took the responsibility himself to put them into effect. In May 1902, dissatisfied with the manner with which the Brisbane Municipal Council was pursuing its role in the campaign, the new commissioner issued an "order" directing the council to do its duty within the time prescribed in the "order". One of Ham's annual reports said a gang of fifty men had been employed for two months during which time some three thousand loads of filth and rubbish were removed from the area, and either jettisoned at sea or destroyed by fire. Despite Ham's efforts, cases of plague continued to occur for the next nine years in Queensland but the incidence was not as high as it had been in 1900. In the decade in which the disease was present in the state there were 499 cases with 219 deaths. The Polynesians were present in Queensland in large numbers for the first half of the decade, after which deportation back to their native islands began. Only two cases occurred in the islanders. The incidence was higher in the Chinese with 22 cases, most of them fatal. But the earlier predictions that they would be found responsible for the epidemic was false. The conditions in many of the places where the white people worked and lived were so conducive for rat breeding that the blame could not be placed elsewhere. Ham did not prove to be a Pied Piper of Hamlin but without his efforts the incidence and the deaths from plague would have been much higher.

There were many tragic cases during the ten years that plague was present in Queensland. A young lad, attracted by the increase from two to six pence in the bounty paid for dead rats began collecting the animals. Instead of making his fortune, he met his death from the disease passed on from the source of his income. Charles Wray, medical officer with the municipal council, contracted the disease while conducting a post-mortem and died in May 1902. A report of a localized outbreak of plague in January 1907 found that "The first six cases were those of schoolboys at home for the holidays, and as playmates were in constant association with each other, up to the time of the attacks." Sixteen people living in the small block bounded by four streets in New Farm, Brisbane, had contracted the disease. There were five deaths. The father of one of the boys kept a general and produce store in James Street in the suburb. It proved to be the source of infection common to all the cases. The boys were in the habit of frequenting the produce shed and helped handle the produce. There was evidence of recent rat infestation in the shed, a history of dead rats having been seen previous to the outbreak. The other victims either lived close to the store or were members of a gang employed in removing "a large accumulation of filth, consisting of animal and vegetable matter, dust and debris from beneath the incriminated general and fruit stores".

Maryborough was the scene of a sub-epidemic in which eight people of nine attacked, five in the one family, died from a different type of the disease. John O'Connell, a lad of seventeen years employed at a fruiterer's shop, became ill on 19 May, and was at home for six days before a doctor was called just prior his death. The cause of death was certified as "pneumonia". John was of a motherless family of seven and had been nursed by a kindly neighbour. She, too, died three days after John's death. She was buried without a death certificate being issued, an action which brought caustic comment from the magistrate at a subsequent inquiry. Four more children in the O'Connell family died with symptoms like those of pneumonia in the Maryborough Hospital. By this time the medical authorities realized that the "pneumonia" could be pneumonic plague in which the plague germs are passed on, not by the bites of fleas, but through inhaling in the manner most chest infections are contracted. Post-mortems of those who died in hospital confirmed this suspicion but not before three of the nursing staff developed the disease. Two of these women died. Further cases were prevented by inoculating the medical and nursing staff of the hospital which was quarantined; the burning of the the O'Connell house and contents and a war on the rat population of Maryborough. A small memorial tablet hanging on the wall near the medical superintendent's office at the Maryborough Hospital is a grim reminder of the tragedy.

Erected in Memory of
Nurses Rose A. Wiles and Cecilia E. Bauer,
Who died whilst devotedly discharging their duty
In the service of the institution
during 1905.

War Hysteria

Brisbane newspapers in the early days of World War I reported that the declaration of war by Britain on Germany roused the populace to a great pitch of patriotic fervour. They told of the large and ever-increasing crowd of enthusiastic citizens forcing the meeting scheduled for the Town Hall to be transferred to Market-square; of the crowd of five thousand greeting the mayor with loud cheering when he spoke of "the scarlet thread of kinship with the mother country, blood of our blood, bone of our bone" and of the spontaneous procession afterwards through the city streets with patriotic songs being sung till lungs were exhausted. An editorial in the *Brisbane Courier* of 6 August 1914, couched in more sober terms, reminded its readers that:

> In this country there are many citizens of German birth and extraction. It is to be deplored that a larrikin element in Melbourne has lately risen up to demonstrate against our German fellow citizens. That does not represent Australian feeling. Germans have come to us and have been admitted to a common citizenship; they have been honest, loyal and honoured. Our war is as between nations, not individuals and no British man or woman worthy of the name should say one word to embitter the hearts of the German people of Australia, who are saddened by the calamity which we share in common.

But as time passed people ignored the exhortations of the *Courier* and an open bitterness towards the Germans in the Australian community developed. Many German men were interned and their wives, often of British stock, were ostracized by former friends, their children taunted with references to their parentage. One of the many families who found themselves in this predicament was that of Dr Eugen Hirschfeld.

Born in 1866 at Mitisch in Silesia, Eugen Hirschfeld followed a family tradition in studying medicine. After a course interrupted in 1886–87 by twelve months' compulsory military service, he graduated from Strasburg University in 1887. Passing the state examination necessary for registration the next year he was then awarded a doctorate in medicine in 1889 after submitting a thesis on the pigments of the eye. He came to Queensland at a time when holders of the state examination of Germany were recognized automatically by the medical board, and was registered in the colony on 7 August 1890. Graduating during a period when his countrymen Robert Koch, Emil Von Behring and Paul Ehrlich were making significant discoveries in the cause and the control of infectious diseases, it is not surprising that Hirschfeld interested himself in the same field when he came to Queensland. He became honorary bacteriologist to the Brisbane Hospital and in the years immediately following his arrival in Queensland contributed many papers to the Royal Society of Queensland and the medical journals. His papers covered the prevention and treatment of infectious diseases generally as well as dealing with specific diseases. In 1892 when the Queensland parliament was debating the leprosy bill he shared the forum at a meeting of the Royal Society of Queensland with the governor of Queensland, Sir Henry Norman. Hirschfeld dealt with the laboratory diagnosis of the disease while His Excellency drew on his experiences with lepers in India and the West Indies. In the same year the German doctor wrote on the organism believed at the time to be the cause of influenza. After a series of epidemics of dengue fever in Queensland he delivered a classic description of the disease to the Intercolonial Medical Congress in 1898. However, Hirschfeld's greatest interest was in tuberculosis, both in cattle and in humans. In 1891 he was cooperating with the Department of Agriculture and Stock in the use of tuberculin — a preparation made from the tuberculosis organism by Robert Koch the year before. Hailed first as a possible cure for the disease it proved to be a useful diagnostic tool. The *Queenslander* referred to Hirschfeld's work in these terms:

> We do, however, rejoice to know that its [tuberculin's] effectiveness is about to be tried upon live stock by a gentleman with so high a scientific reputation as that of Dr Hirschfeld.

Three years later he advocated the inspection of meat by trained meat inspectors to look for tuberculosis and other diseases. Much of his work with tuberculosis in humans was performed at the Diamantina Hospital for Chronic Diseases at South Brisbane. When the doctor went overseas in 1912, the Queensland government requested him to study the latest advances in the treatment of tuberculosis. The value of his report on his return became known to the New South Wales government which asked for a complete copy. In addition to being honorary bacteriologist to the Brisbane Hospital he was also an honorary physician to the institution. Whilst his services were employed

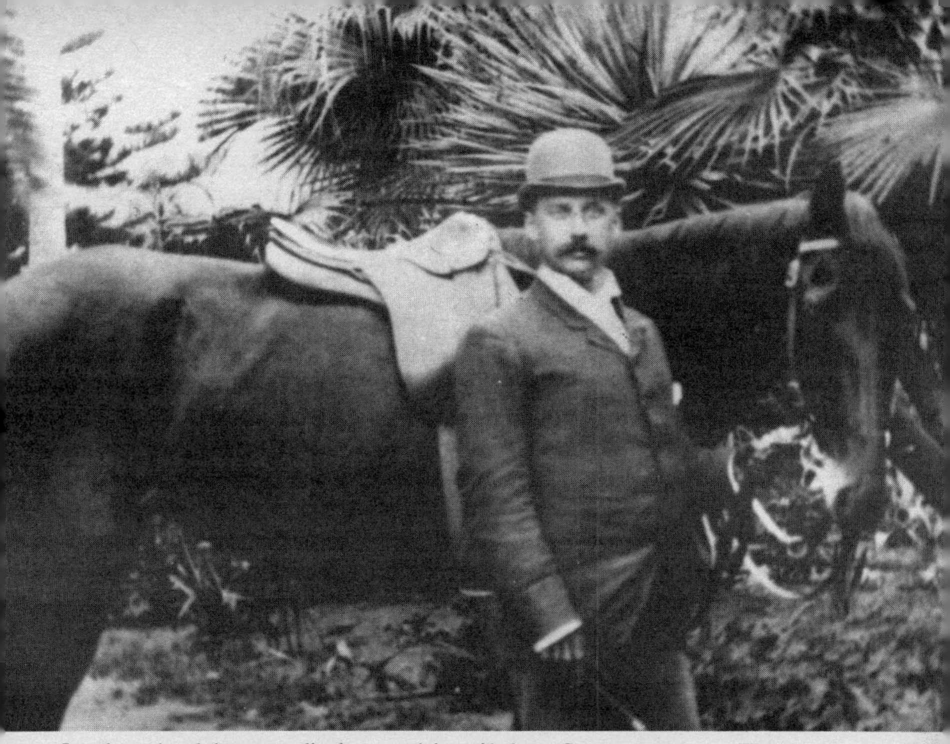

Imprisoned and then extradited on suspicion of being a German spy during World War I, Dr Eugen Hirschfeld (pictured around 1908) fought the government and the medical profession for justice. (Courtesy Dr Konrad Hirschfeld)

generally he spent much of his time at the hospital caring for typhoid patients who were filling the fever wards during his term of office. It was not surprising that a practitioner with his record was appointed to the Medical Board of Queensland.

Hirschfeld became a naturalized British subject in 1893 but maintained his German citizenship by registering with the German consul in Brisbane, Von Ploennes, in 1900. The legal consequences of this action were later to be disputed. He married an Australian girl, Anne, daughter of V.J. Saddler of Melbourne, in 1896. There were four surviving children from the marriage and two sons, Otto and Konrad, kept up the family tradition of studying medicine. In 1906 Hirschfeld succeeded Von Ploennes as German consul for Queensland. In his capacity as consul he gave a dinner in honour of the German emperor's birthday in January 1907 which was attended by several members of the Queensland cabinet. The new consul suggested to his superior in Sydney in 1908 that four German doctors, including himself, examine German reservists in Queensland in lieu of the previous practice of their being examined by doctors on warships visiting Australia. He also encouraged his fellow countrymen in

Queensland to maintain the German language and traditions. When the University of Queensland was established Hirschfeld was appointed a member of the university senate and the institution later honoured him by conferring on him an honorary doctorate of medicine. At a congress of British universities held in London in 1912 the doctor represented the University of Queensland with Sir Robert Philip and Sir Thomas Robinson. In July 1914 he was one of seven new members appointed to the Queensland Legislative Council. The Labour newspaper, the *Daily Standard*, claimed the others were a fine collection of stolid old Tories but considered Dr Hirschfeld was the pick of the bunch, saying that he was a good man, clear from the dust of violent prejudice. He took his seat in the upper house on 7 July, just four weeks before the outbreak of the war.

On 7 August the *Brisbane Courier* made the following reference to the German consul in Brisbane.

> By virtue of the declaration of war communication between the State and the German Consul automatically ceases. Dr Hirschfeld for something like 8 years has held this responsible position in Queensland with conspicuous success and ability and the international relationships have been maintained with both dignity and friendliness. That Dr Hirschfeld's efforts have been appreciated in high quarters as well as by the general public is illustrated by the following memorandum which was issued last night by the Premier, Hon. D.F. Denham.
>
> International law prescribes that the functions and appointment of a consul cease on a declaration of war. Accordingly Dr Hirschfeld is now no longer German Consul. Dr Hirschfeld has discharged the duties of German Consul for eight years, during which term of office he has not only won the confidence and the thanks of his countrymen but he has ever impressed on his countrymen the duty of loyalty to the country of their adoption.

During October 1914 reports of atrocities allegedly committed by the Germans in Belgium appeared in the Brisbane press. There were references to "rape, mutilation, lust and frenzy of drink by the maddened soldiery" and claims that "the whole of Belgium has been given over to the passions of maddened men". Allegedly "a village was fired and all the inhabitants thrown into the flames". Such accounts embittered the Brisbane people and Hirschfeld was caught up in that bitterness, the first overt evidence of which was revealed in parliament. After a number of questions asked at intervals by Thomas Welsby, member for Merthyr, about the matter of Hirschfeld's retention of membership of the Legislative Council, the subject came to a head at the beginning of November 1914. Extracts from Hansard read as follows:

> Mr Williams (Charters Towers) asked the Treasurer, in the absence of the Premier —
> "1. Is he aware that the retention by Dr Hirschfeld of his seat in the Legislative Council is causing widespread dissatisfaction and uneasiness in the State?
> "2. As Dr Hirschfeld has not resigned his seat in the Council, will he introduce or support a Bill in Parliament, having for its object the removal of Dr Hirschfeld from the Legislative Council, or will he take other steps to alleviate the position?"
> The Treasurer (Hon. W.H. Barnes, Bulimba) replied —
> "1 and 2. Shortly after the outbreak of war Dr Hirschfeld intimated to the Chief Secretary that if his retention of a seat in the Legislative Council embarrassed, or was likely to embarrass, the Government, he would resign. It was not suggested, on either side, that in such event the Government would call on him to do so. More recently, Dr Hirschfeld has, without any suggestion from the Government, come to the conclusion that such retention might cause embarrassment, and consequently, on Saturday last, he addressed a letter to the Chief Secretary stating that he had handed his resignation as a member of the Legislative Council to the Lieutenant-Governor. The Government desire to place on record in 'Votes and Proceedings' that since his appointment Dr Hirschfeld has done nothing by word or deed to justify his being regarded as other than a loyal Queensland citizen, or as a worthy member of the Legislative Council. I should like to add that as Senior Honorary Physician to the General and Mater Misericordiae Hospitals, and as a Senator of the University of Queensland, and in other capacities, Dr Hirschfeld has rendered good service to the community."

While the Treasurer expressed his belief in Hirschfeld's loyalty there were many in the community who did not agree with him and the medical profession was one group to reveal it openly. Reflecting hostility engendered by the publication of growing casualty lists of Australians who had landed at Gallipoli in April 1915, the Queensland branch of the British Medical Association called a special meeting on 14 May to discuss Hirschfeld's membership. The president, Archibald Brockway, told the members present that there were no rules to deal with such a position but that it was war and the matter should be dealt with accordingly. Dr Hirschfeld had shown his sympathy with the enemy by giving a dinner party on the kaiser's birthday although he was a British subject. It was resolved that Dr Hirschfeld be asked to resign. If he failed to do so his name would be struck from the list of members. Dr Hirschfeld obliged. But the doctors were not yet satisfied. At a further meeting a week later, George Hopkins drew attention to the recent reappointment of Dr Hirschfeld to the honorary staff of the Brisbane Hospital and he added that he did not consider that other members of the staff should be asked to work with him. Despite efforts to persuade the hospital committee to ask Dr Hirschfeld to resign, his appointment was continued till the end of 1915.

Meanwhile Hirschfeld was being kept under surveillance by army intelligence officers and they reported in December 1915:

> He (Hirschfeld) is a very cute person and is spoken a lot of by the British residents of the town but nothing can be obtained against him. He is very closely watched and his correspondence is strictly censored.

The censor reported:

> With regard to Dr Hirschfeld (late German Consul), I have to state that beyond a few business letters in connection with his practice and a few addressed to his wife (who I understand is an English woman) nothing of consequence goes to him through the post.

But in the community wild rumours circulated. It was alleged that he had known the war was being planned eighteen years before, and that at every confinement he had attended where a male child was born he had maimed the baby in such a way that he would not be fit for military duty when he grew up. Another rumour claimed that the German doctor was responsible for an epidemic of meningitis at the Enoggera army camp by injecting Australian soldiers with the meningitis germs. Army intelligence officers found no subversive actions being committed by Hirschfeld but weight of public opinion influenced George Pearce, the minister for Defence, to sign a warrant for his internment on 11 February 1916 which was executed a few days later. Part of the warrant read:

> AND WHEREAS in the opinion of the Minister for securing the public safety and the defence of the Commonwealth it is expedient in view of the hostile origin and associations of E. Hirschfeld, of Brisbane in the state of Queensland that he should be detained in military custody during the continuance of the present war.
>
> NOW THEREFORE, I, George Foster Pearce, Minister of State for Defence do hereby order that the said E. Hirschfeld shall be detained during the continuance of the present state of war in military custody in some place appointed for the accommodation of persons detained in military custody.

> Provided that any representations against this order by the said E. Hirschfeld shall be forthwith transmitted to and will be duly considered by me.

Hirschfeld's representations against the order, admitting his origin in Germany but denying any hostile associations, were to no avail and he was taken to the Trial Bay internment camp, at the mouth of the Macleay River, near Kempsey, New South Wales.

Originally a gaol built in the latter half of the nineteenth century, it had ceased to function as a prison in 1903 and was acquired by the Australian army in 1915. The internees at Trial Bay came mainly from the professions, or business and executive positions. From the prison, sited on a headland, they could roam over several acres of land down to the sea, where swimming was permitted. But it was still an internment camp. Hirschfeld, not surprisingly, made several attempts to be released. Efforts were also made for the release of Carl Zoeller, a naturalized British subject with a cutlery and medical instrument business in Queen Street, Brisbane. Hearing of these efforts, the commandant of the First Military District in Queensland wrote to headquarters in Melbourne:

> Information has come before me that the question of the release of Messrs Hirschfeld and Zoeller has again been raised.
>
> The feeling against both of these persons is exceptionally pronounced in the District and their release would cause such dissatisfaction throughout Queensland as would considerably nullify the beneficial effects of all internments.
>
> Both Hirschfeld and Zoeller are men of position, and their release would be considered to have been effected by their means and influence.

However, Hirschfeld was released on medical grounds in August 1917, and was allowed to return to his home on Wickham Terrace, Brisbane, where he was kept under strict military guard — for which he was obliged to pay. Five weeks later he was examined by Lieutenant Colonel Joseph Espie Dods who "failed to discover any medical reason that should prevent him being interned in either a camp or hospital for internees provided there is a resident medical officer attached to the camp or hospital" and Hirschfeld found himself back at Trial Bay. Early in 1917 the army had received advice that German sympathizers in Java intended to mount an expedition to rescue internees at Trial Bay. This report was ignored, but in 1918 it was learnt that the

German raider, *Wolf*, had visited the New South Wales coast, and a decision was made to close Trial Bay. The internees were transferred to Liverpool camp, which had been established in 1914. At times there were five thousand internees at Liverpool and conditions were less congenial than those at Trial Bay.

The end of the war in November 1918 brought no mass release of internees. The Australian government was giving consideration to their deportation and Hirschfeld waited his fate at Liverpool along with thousands of others. He was there in the early months of 1919 when the epidemic of influenza reached Australia. The concentration camp did not escape the epidemic and at the request of the camp commandant Dr Hirschfeld organized and supervised a 250-bed fever hospital, declining any reward for his services. As happened elsewhere there were a number of deaths from the disease among the internees. In May 1919 Mrs Hirschfeld received the disturbing news from the military authorities in Queensland that her husband might be deported. Being a British subject herself, she and her children would be permitted to remain in Australia. This advice led to increased efforts to prevent Hirschfeld's being sent out of the country. However, the authorities could now produce evidence which they believed would tell against the former consul. The German consul's files, which had been in bond at His Majesty's Customs for the duration of the war, were now in the hands of army intelligence in Brisbane. Documents in the German language were translated by Johannes Tilanus, attached to the army intelligence section. Tilanus's report contained three charges against Hirschfeld. He was accused of encouraging "Germanism" in Queensland by advocating the speaking of the German language by his fellow countrymen and the maintenance of German traditions; of secretly renouncing his British naturalization by his registering with the German consul in 1900, thus reverting to a German national; and of being connected with the German army. Evidence of the last two charges was allegedly contained in a letter written by Hirschfeld in German in July 1908 to the German consul general in Sydney. He had suggested that four German doctors living in Queensland conduct examinations of German reservists in the state instead of the previous practice of their being examined when German warships carrying doctors visited Australian ports. The sentence which supposedly demonstrated his guilt was: "Vier reichsdeutsche aerzte sind in Queensland wohnhaft Dr P. Heymann (Lowood), Dr Hinrichsen (Toowoomba), Dr Martschk (Brisbane) und ich selbst." The key word is *reichsdeutsche* — a German national. An acceptable translation of the sentence is: "There are four doctors who are German nationals residing in Queensland, namely Dr P. Heymann (Lowood), Dr Hinrichsen (Toowoomba), Dr Martschk (Brisbane) and myself." Tilanus was translating at the end of the war and he was fully aware of the swell of public opinion against Hirschfeld. He gave the meaning of "unnaturalized" to reichsdeutsche, implying that by placing his name on the consul's register Hirschfeld had secretly renounced his naturalization as a British citizen. The former consul later strongly denied this, claiming that it was legal for a person to hold citizenship of two countries simultaneously — an opinion supported by legal advice. However, Tilanus's translation was accepted and passed up the chain of command without even the highest official questioning it in any way. Further, the interpreter passed judgment on Hirschfeld as well as translating the documents. This, too, was accepted by superior officers. Part of Tilanus's report reads as follows:

> These latter [documents] are of great importance because they show the activities of the German Consul at Brisbane, furnishing ample proof that the German Consul overstepped his sphere of action as a Consul, as laid down by International law and usage, and how he acted as an agent of the German Government and used or misused his official position to found a German State in Queensland. . .
>
> The whole of the correspondence proves Dr Hirschfeld was a most unscrupulous man, and it furnishes proof of intended invasion of Australia as outlined in my report on Prisoner of War, Ronald Gordon.

(Ronald Gordon made a fictitious claim that he had information of the plans of a Power A to invade Australia, and was deported.) Captain Cyril Wood of the army intelligence section, Brisbane, was the first officer to accept Tilanus's translation and opinion and did not shift his ground even when he received legal opinion on the documents. When requested by Wood for an opinion, Brisbane solicitors Chambers and McNab indicated that under Australian law as existed at the time it was in order for a person to hold double citizenship. Their advice was:

> Certain papers have been submitted to us being translations of documents which came from the possession of Dr Hirschfeld, and our opinion has been asked as to whether he has been guilty of any criminal offence.
>
> It appears from the papers that prior to the War one of the chief aims of the German pastors was to keep alive the German language and the love of Germany amongst the various colonies of Germans in

> Queensland, even to the second generation of those born in Australia and Dr Hirschfeld was instrumental in obtaining a so-called honorarium for these pastors.
>
> It also appears that the German reservists were in the habit of being medically examined on board a German man-of-war, on its periodical visits to Australia and in 1908 Dr Hirschfeld as German Consul suggested the appointment of four German doctors in Queensland to examine Germans liable for military service.
>
> In one letter written to a German in Charters Towers, he says — "I may call your attention to the fact that your naturalisation in Australia does not debar you from being at the same time of German nationality if you become naturalised for the purpose of obtaining property", and informs him how he can apply for re-admission into the Prussian States Union.
>
> It seems to be recognised that a person can be a subject of two countries at the same time. (See Notes on Nationality Manual of War Precautions, 7th Edition page 248.)
>
> All the events covered by the documents happened some years before the War, and although they might raise a suspicion that there was some ulterior object for preserving the German language and nationality, there is nothing that would amount to a criminal offence.
>
> Dr Hirschfeld having been re-naturalised as a German subject after having been naturalised as a British subject, would not in our opinion render him liable to criminal proceedings.

Captain Wood also sent copies of the documents to the Department of Defence, Melbourne, asking "whether a naturalised British subject of German descent commits an act of High Treason when he takes the oath of allegiance to the Kaiser and so becomes a German subject again as provided for in German law". Wood must have been disappointed with the reply from the Department of Defence that it was "doubtful whether any criminal offence has been committed by Dr Hirschfeld".

In July 1919 there was a rather sinister turn in the affair. Tilanus, the interpreter, stole some of the documents from the German consul files. With Philip Holzberger, a Brisbane solicitor, he went to Mrs Hirschfeld. Telling her that without the papers the authorities would not be able to deport her husband, he offered them to her for £200. Mrs Hirschfeld consulted her solicitors and took the matter to the Defence department. Tilanus and Holzberger were charged with conspiracy. Holzberger was sentenced to three months imprisonment with hard labour and fined £200. A sentence of two years imprisonment with hard labour imposed on Tilanus was suspended under the first offenders section of the criminal code and he was set free on a good behaviour bond.

Hundreds of internees were deported but still Hirschfeld waited in Liverpool camp. However, in November 1919 he returned to Brisbane on parole. His appearance triggered a storm of protests. The *Daily Mail* reported one demonstration under the headline "DEPORT HIM AT ONCE".

> About 2,000 soldiers, discharged soldiers and sympathisers met in Albert square last night, and carried, amid enthusiasm, a resolution demanding the immediate deportation of Dr Hirschfeld.
>
> Mr Montefiore, who presided, said: "I am not certain whether all here are aware of the fact, but it is a solemn truth that Dr Hirschfeld has been released from the internment camp and is walking about tonight — a free man. (Uproar) I say that it is enough to make a soldier's blood boil."
>
> A Digger: We'll fix him.
>
> Another Digger: Leave him to us. We'll be up there.
>
> Mr Montefiore: The resolution I have to move is this:- "That this meeting of returned soldiers and citizens demands the immediate deportation of Dr Hirschfeld from Australia and his return to Germany".
>
> Sandford Jackson, a prominent Brisbane medico and president of the King and Empire Alliance sent this telegram to Prime Minister Hughes.
>
> In the absence of any particulars either as to the reason for the internment of Dr Hirschfeld or for his release and return to this city, public opinion in Brisbane is in a state of ferment. Excitement and indignation are being freely expressed and much harm is being done to the cause of loyalty. We suggest an immediate public statement by you.

The prime minister also received a copy of a resolution from the Queensland branch of the British Medical Association which had been introduced by John Lockhart Gibson and David Hardie. It read:

> As it is impossible to doubt that there must have been sufficient reason for the internment of Dr Hirschfeld, we are of the opinion that the generous treatment accorded to him in this community prior to the war, accentuates enormously any disloyalty he may have shown and accentuates also the necessity for his deportation.

The protests led to Hirschfeld's arrest and return to the Liverpool internment camp. With his fate still undecided he was again released on parole in January 1920 in Sydney. Once again the opposing bodies made loud protestations, with the Queensland branch of the British Medical Association influencing the federal council of the association to ask the commonwealth government to deport all medical practitioners of enemy origin who had been interned during the war.

In March 1920 Hirschfeld appeared before an aliens board consisting of C.F. Butler, a Sydney magistrate as chairman, Captain Wood of the Queensland army intelligence section and Captain Wallace from the New South Wales section. There were no formal charges but he was questioned about his connection with the German army by examining German reservists, about his renaturalization as a German citizen and his fostering the German language and traditions. Butler's report to Pearce, the minister for Defence, was devastating. The magistrate recommended the doctor's compulsory repatriation, saying:

> If this applicant is allowed to remain in the Commonwealth in my opinion he would be dangerous to the State on account of his influence and special qualifications. . .
>
> I am fully convinced that Hirschfeld is a person whose conduct clearly shows that he considered himself to be a subject of Germany and that at all available opportunities he did everything in his power to foster the German national spirit, thereby conclusively proving his disaffection to the British Empire after he had given his Oath of Allegiance.

Pearce approved the recommendation but requested the solicitor general, Sir Robert Garran, to comment on the legality of the intended action. Garran's advice indicates that he, too, accepted the original translation of the letter of July 1908 in which Hirschfeld had suggested four German doctors examine German reservists and that he also believed Hirschfeld had renounced his British naturalization. He said:

> It appears that Dr Hirschfeld was naturalised in Queensland, but the Stipendiary Magistrate's report states that he admits that in 1900 he registered himself at the German Consulate, Brisbane, as a German citizen. This is borne out by papers on the file.
>
> Moreover, in a letter of 27 July 1908, to the German Consul-General, Sydney, he described himself as an *unnaturalised* German doctor — in which capacity he places himself at the disposal of the German Foreign Office for the examination in Queensland of men due for German military service. In my opinion, Dr Hirschfeld has clearly brought himself under the Aliens' Restriction Order.

Shortly after his appearance before the aliens board, the *Medical Journal of Australia* carried an editorial which may have been appropriate at the time but when read sixty years later does not seem worthy of that journal.

Some of the Germans practising before 1914 in our chief cities laid claims to special knowledge and special skill, but in no single instance was the verdict of the best judges, the medical practitioners themselves, favourable. In Brisbane, Dr Eugen Hirschfeld was admitted to many positions of importance not because of his eminence in his profession, but for other reasons. He was a member of the Medical Board under a deplorably antiquated Medical Act. He was accorded most generous treatment by the Brisbane practitioners and was accepted as a colleague.

It is stated that he secured his temporary release on the plea of ill-health. It is further stated that this alleged ill-health was based on the presence of albumin in his urine, but the albumin was derived from the poultry farm. . .

We have a right to claim in Australia that those whose conduct was disloyal to the King and Country shall not be allowed to worm themselves in between the men who served and their erstwhile patients. There is no sound argument in favour of being magnanimous to those who rejoiced when the enemy seemingly gained a temporary advantage over our troops, who gloated over the sinking of the Lusitania and who made themselves hateful to the people of their adopted country. There is only one reply to such flagrant abuse of frank and kindly hospitality. They must be turned adrift somewhere — anywhere beyond the confines of the sunny Commonwealth. We have no space for them here.

Despite the sentiments expressed in the journal, influential men, headed by Hirschfeld's father-in-law, Saddler, were endeavouring to have the decision reversed. General, Sir John Monash, probably Australia's greatest soldier, wrote to Garran on Hirschfeld's behalf. Although indebted to Saddler for his start in life, Monash was not the type of man to take up unworthy causes. His letter reads:

Mr V.J. Saddler who is a very old friend of mine, and to whom more than any other man, I owe the help which he gave me in my career, has asked me to write to you to solicit your sympathetic interest in the case of Dr Hirschfeld, a Queensland internee, who is his son-in-law. It happens that I knew Dr Hirschfeld, his wife and family very well before the War, and should be very surprised indeed if there were in existence any tangible evidence of this man's disloyalty to British interests. Quite the contrary. Few men of German descent whom I have known have identified themselves more closely and helpfully with Australian life, or have given more definite evidence of a desire permanently to embrace Australian nationality.

There is indeed some reason in this case to suspect persecution by the very junior military officers who have hitherto dealt with the case.

> I have read some papers in the matter, and Hirschfeld's attitude strikes me as in every way satisfactory, frank and manly.
>
> I do not think that it can be the policy of the Government, now that the War is over, to favour anything in the nature of persecution of an unfortunate man, or, by ordering his deportation, to bring misery to a number of worthy Australian people. I feel very oppressed by this case, and sincerely hope that no factor is present in it which would preclude a lenient decision.

Two Queensland politicians took up Hirschfeld's cause with the minister for Defence. Randolph Bedford, a member of the Legislative Council said this in his letter:

> Australia cannot afford to be guilty of this cruel injustice. If it be confirmed, Mrs Hirschfeld and her children must either bid farewell to their husband and father or they must lose their right to live in their own country, and must abandon that citizenship which is theirs by right of birth. It is useless to say that a just tribunal has recommended it — we don't know that it has any more justice or good sense than any other star chamber preceding it, and the evidence should know only one place of receipt, and that an open Court and before an Australian jury.

Arnold Weinholt, a big game hunter with a distinguished war record, represented the electorate of Moreton in the commonwealth parliament. He was dissatisfied with "just an examination before a naturally prejudiced tribunal and wanted Hirschfeld to have a fair opportunity to answer the charges against him". He added: "I wish to state quite openly I am not at all convinced now of Hirschfeld's having done anything disloyal. I am not in the slightest concerned with the deportation of any German Aliens; nor do I consider anyone has any cause for complaint against internment." Wienholt incurred the wrath of the Returned Servicemen's League (today known as the RSL) by his actions. However, his representations together with other pressures succeeded in delaying the deportation and in having the minister for Defence ask Garran, the solicitor general, to carefully review the case. As a result, the press announced that Dr Hirschfeld and Father Jerger were not in a group of Germans who left Sydney on the steamer *Main* on 5 June, as was expected. Father Jerger had attracted the attention of the authorities when members of his congregation at St Brigid's Roman Catholic Church alleged that the priest expressed his disloyalty to the British empire during his services. The two men were the subjects of demonstrations in the Sydney Domain organized by the Loyal Orange Institute of

New South Wales. Press reports of the delay in Hirschfeld's deportation again sparked off emotional protests in Brisbane. In an hysterical outburst at a branch meeting of the Returned Servicemen's League, the president said: "To my mind he is guilty of the greatest crime on this earth, and that is being a German. Certainly he is not responsible for that, but it is a crime and ought to be put at the head of the Criminal Code."

Hirschfeld was interrogated by Garran in Sydney on 10 June 1920. Again there were no formal charges but the enquiry was based on the previous allegations dealing with the questions of naturalization, the fostering of "Germanism" and the medical examination of German reservists. The solicitor general seemed to place much importance on the letter written by Hirschfeld dealing with the examination of reservists, for he asked several questions centred on it. Hirschfeld must have had great difficulty recalling what he had written twelve years previously and he was not permitted to see the documents. After Garran offered no comment to the former consul's assertion that double citizenship was well known and not illegal the questions and answers were as follows:

> Garran. — Well, some years six years later, it was in 1908, you described yourself to the Consul General in Sydney as an "Unnaturalised German doctor", as one of four unnaturalised German doctors.
> Hirschfeld. — That is a falsehood absolutely. I was Consul at the time and would not state a palpable lie. They knew by my appointment that I was naturalised.
> Garran. — The translation of a letter dated 22nd July 1908 says: — "The examination of men due for military service is to take place in Queensland . . . Four unnaturalised German doctors reside in Queensland, namely [—] and my self. I have requested all these gentlemen to place themselves at the disposal of the Foreign Office".
> Hirschfeld. — I absolutely could have no interest in making a statement like that because they knew when I was appointed Consul that I was naturalised. I am quite certain I could not have written a note like that, because I always have described myself as a naturalised British Queensland subject. I would like to see the Register, Sir, because I am not such a fool as to tell a lie when they knew by my description that I was naturalised.

At the conclusion of the interrogation Garran promised to go through the papers and have them checked where there was any doubt but he reported to the prime minister that he saw no reason to alter the previous decision that Hirschfeld should be deported.

The battle was over and Hirschfeld left Australia in September 1920. His wife and children stayed in Australia. The children had reached important stages in their education with one son, Otto, now studying medicine at Melbourne University. During his deportation period Dr Hirschfeld practised medicine at Allantown, Pennsylvannia, in the United States. In 1923 Monash again took up his cudgels, writing unsuccessfully to S.M. Bruce who was now the prime minister. However in 1926 further efforts were rewarded and J.G. Latham, the attorney general, reviewed the case and allowed Hirschfeld to return to Australia. He found that during his long absence his wife had carefully supervised their children's progress. Otto had completed his medical course and was beginning what turned out to be a most successful career. Just prior to his father's return Konrad, also at Melbourne University studying medicine, had been awarded a Rhodes Scholarship.

General Monash, anticipating opposition from the returned soldiers in Queensland, wrote to Major Maddock. Monash's attitude in the matter can be seen from the following extracts.

> I am writing to you on a matter of some delicacy, viz. the case of Dr Hirschfeld.
>
> I feel sure that you will be quite ready to accept my assurance that there is a great deal in the circumstances surrounding this case which has never been made public.
>
> If it were true that Hirschfeld had done nothing to justify his permanent banishment from his family and from the home of his adoption, then I feel that an injustice has been done even more poignant and inhuman than in the famous case of Captain Dreyfus in France some years ago.
>
> The present Attorney General, Mr Latham, was induced recently to look personally into the files of the case, and had no difficulty in coming to the conclusion that there was no justification for the continuance of such an inhuman and unjust state of affairs, and accordingly the Federal Government has given permission for Hirschfeld to rejoin his family.
>
> You must be perfectly well aware that I would be the last man in the world to sanction any action which would permit of treachery or anything of that nature being countenanced in this country, but the days of war hysteria are now over, and one should bring to bear upon such a question a spirit of fair play and charity. If, as I believe, this man is not guilty of any other crime than of having been born a German and having made Australia the home of his permanent adoption, it would be assuredly a wicked thing, of which the Australian nation ought to be well ashamed, if a decree of banishment were to persisted in.

> I notice with some concern that the Brisbane Branch of the League has been taking this matter up, and therefore thought that perhaps an expression of opinion by myself would weigh with them.

Monash's hope that his opinion would weigh with the Brisbane returned soldiers was not realized. After the prime minister addressed a Brisbane meeting about referendum proposals he was bombarded about the reason for Hirschfeld's return. At a public meeting of the Returned Servicemen's League in the School of Arts in Ann Street, Brisbane, Thomas Welsby, who presided, said that "it was a crying cruel shame permitting him to return". Cyril Wood, the former intelligence officer, was one of the main speakers. He regretted that his oath of secrecy prevented him from producing a document which would convince the prime minister that "that man would never again come into Australia". However, their protests were in vain.

The former consul, now sixty years of age, practised medicine for a few years and then purchased a property at Bybera on the Darling Downs where "his scientific and practical contributions to rural science were as outstanding as was his work in the fields of public health and medicine in the prewar years". His work in this area so impressed the premier, Frank Cooper, that in January 1945 he invited him to address the cabinet, other members of the Legislative Assembly and senior government officers on "Queensland Pastures; Their Development and Improvement". He died at the age of eighty in 1947. Otto Hirschfeld became a highly respected physician and chancellor of the University of Queensland. The youngest son, Konrad, specialized in surgery with the same success and served on the senate of the university for many years. In 1978 Konrad was awarded the CBE for services to medicine and education. When he was further honoured by the university in 1982 with an honorary doctorate of medicine over fifty colleagues recognized the award by feting him with a dinner.

The Bundaberg Tragedy

> The entire city of Bundaberg was in deep mourning yesterday, when the last tribute was paid to child victims of the fatal injections of anti-diphtheria serum. Bundaberg has never passed through such a grief-stricken period. Women and children wept in the streets, and strong men were moved to tears as the tiny coffins passed by. The scenes at the graveside were unforgettable. . . The whole city came to a stand-still, business houses and hotels closed their doors, and people flocked into the streets in thousands to pay their last sad tributes of respect to the innocent victims.
>
> Shortly after 10 o'clock the dull thud of muffled drums, and the mournful music of the bands struck up and continued at intervals for the rest of the day.
>
> The fourth funeral which took place at 2.15 was one that moved the seething mass of humanity to tears. The main street was thronged and the deathly silence was broken only by the sobbing of the vast multitude as the little white coffins passed by. . . Terrible was the scene as the remains of three bonny boys (from one family) who had played together and brightened the home of their devoted parents passed enroute to their resting place.

The above extracts from the *Brisbane Courier* of 30 January 1928 depict the harrowing scenes that followed what is known in public health circles as "The Bundaberg Tragedy". In an editorial in the same issue the *Courier* said that, "Throughout the whole Commonwealth the deepest sympathy will be felt for those bereaved and stricken parents at Bundaberg who, in a desire to save their children from a dreaded epidemic of diphtheria saw them die from the very remedy that should have saved them". The events that led up to the tragedy had been reported in the paper the day before:

> The campaign for the immunisation of children against diphtheria has led to a terrible tragedy at Bundaberg owing to a cause which as yet is inexplicable. On Friday last, 19 children received injections of the toxin-antitoxin, six receiving their final treatment, and 13 their first injection. Hitherto no ill effects had followed these operations, but during Friday night some of the patients became ill, with violent attacks of vomiting and diarrhoea. On Saturday morning a number of children were found to be seriously ill, and were hurried to hospital.

> Despite all that medical skill could do, many of the little patients failed to rally, and up to last night 12 deaths had occurred, while five others are dangerously ill. . . "This sad occurrence, which evokes the deepest sympathy for the bereaved parents, is utterly abnormal in the history of this valuable method of preventive treatment," said Dr. J.S. Elkington, Commonwealth Health Department, in an interview yesterday.

Official records indicate that twenty-one children were injected, not nineteen as reported by the *Courier*.

An ancient disease, diphtheria was described by the famous Greek physician, Aretaeus, in a Roman province of Asia Minor, in the second century A.D. Starting as a sore throat, it can kill in two ways. In the throat it forms a membrane which, creeping from the tonsils, can close the windpipe thus suffocating the victim, usually a young child. The Italians aptly called the disease, *garotillo* — the strangler. It also produces a toxin or poison, which, circulating in the body, may produce severe complications in the heart and nervous system. There was a great upsurge of diphtheria in the middle of the nineteenth century and epidemics occurred in many countries, including Australia. For sixty years before the Bundaberg tragedy, there were frequent epidemics in Queensland with the severest mortality in the 1870s. The disease continued to ravage the children in the colony. In 1890 Jefferis Turner, the first full-time resident medical officer at the Brisbane Children's Hospital, told members of the Queensland Medical Society that "By far the worse scourge of children in this city, is diphtheria, from which fifty deaths were recorded during the first six months of this year." Turner went on to say that he could not recommend any treatment for the disease except the surgical opening of the windpipe when the membrane threatened to cut off the air supply to the patient. However a few years later he introduced treatment with antitoxin, which the German scientist, Emil Von Behring, had discovered. It reduced the mortality considerably but some children continued to die from the disease. There was still no prevention and the old diphtheria ward at the Children's Hospital and the isolation wards in Queensland country hospitals were often full with young patients. In 1909 a new diphtheria ward was built at the Children's Hospital — called the Courier Ward as the newspaper had been instrumental in raising much of the funds needed for its erection. The foundation stone was laid by the Earl of Dudley, the governor general of Australia, on 23 August and the ward was ready for occupation three months later. When Sir William MacGregor, performing his first official task after taking up the position of governor of Queensland, opened it on 8 December, he said that in 1908 there had been 150 children in the hospital suffering from the disease and 200 in the current year. The new ward was often full during epidemics. In 1921 there were over 2,400 cases of diphtheria reported in the state, of whom 112, mainly children under the age of five years, died from the disease.

Meanwhile scientists had been studying possible methods of prevention. The first efficient agent produced was a mixture of toxin and an antitoxin. The diphtheria poison was safely neutralized by its anti-poison but the mixture produced protective antibodies when injected. With so many cases of diphtheria occurring and reports of the new product's safety and efficiency it was not surprising that John Moore, the public health commissioner for Queensland, recommended that it should be used by local authorities. The councils were slow to adopt Moore's advice. However, in 1926, two medical officers of health, Mervyn Paterson at Ipswich and Albert Parry at Rockhampton, pioneered immunization against diphtheria with no ill-effects. During 1927 doctors at the Brisbane Children's Hospital immunized over one thousand children and one hundred nurses with no serious reactions. Towards the end of that year Harold Tilling began a campaign for the Brisbane City Council and no complaints of sickness following the injections were received. About this time the Bundaberg City Council decided to follow suit and asked their medical officer of health, Ewing Thomson, to make the necessary arrangements. Thomson, a Sydney graduate of 1910, ordered the toxin-antitoxin mixture, made by the Commonwealth Serum Laboratories early in January 1928. It came in a rubber-capped bottle containing enough immunizing fluid to treat many children. The doctor stored it in an instrument cupboard in his surgery where it was kept in the periods between the injections he made from it. The first injections were performed at the Bundaberg City Council chambers on 17 January 1928. The fluid was drawn from the bottle by puncturing the rubber cap with a needle and the same bottle was used on three more occasions, during one of which his own son received an injection. There were no untoward reactions from the injections on these four occasions. At 4 p.m. on 27 January, twenty-one children from fifteen months to nine years of age received injections. Of these, eight received their first treatment and thirteen a second and larger dose. During the night of 27 January and the early hours of the next morning eighteen children developed similar symptoms and appeared very ill. One child died while being taken to Dr Egmont Schmidt's surgery. Another was admitted to St Vincent's private hospital and fourteen children arrived in close succession at the Bundaberg General Hospital where they were quickly admitted. The sudden arrival of so many desperately sick children was too much for the superintendent, Dr Ivan Hains, to cope with and he sent for help. His colleagues, Ewing Thomson, Leonard McKeown and Samuel Robinson, hurried to the hospital to help. The doctors did all they could for the little victims who were obviously suffering from what was called at the time "blood poisoning". In most cases their efforts were in vain. In all, twelve children died, most of them within twenty-four hours of the injections. Antibiotics were not available in 1928 but the infection was so virulent that even these modern drugs might not have stopped its rapid progress. Specialist services were not available in Bundaberg at the time but it is doubtful whether expert medical assistance could have done other than stand by and confirm that the children were dangerously ill. Three families lost more than one member. The deaths of three boys in one family left the parents childless and two further families were deprived of two daughters and two sons respectively.

Dr Thomson notified the Queensland public health commissioner John Moore, and the commonwealth director general of health, John Cumpston, as soon as he realized the immunizing agent could be involved in the tragedy and both arranged for medical experts to visit the city to investigate the calamity. Dr Earle Page, the commonwealth treasurer, went to Bundaberg to study the events on behalf of his government. The bottle containing the remainder of the fluid used for the injections was handed over for analysis and all the bottles of the same batch were recalled from various parts of Australia. Many had already been used without any serious reactions. Instructions were issued that no more toxin-antitoxin serum was to be issued until the matter had been fully investigated and John Moore ordered the cessation of all immunization programmes in Queensland. The commonwealth government immediately appointed a royal commission to enquire into the tragedy. Its members were Dr Charles Kellaway, director of the Walter and Eliza Hall Institute of Medical Research, Melbourne, Professor Peter McCallum, of Melbourne University, and Dr A.H. Tebbutt, bacteriologist at the University of Sydney.

In the days following the tragedy there were many comments in the press and expression of opinion as to the possible cause. Dr Schmidt, who conducted post-mortem examinations on the victims, said that the cause of the tragedy was a matter of surmise but he agreed that the only explanation was that "latent properties of the serum had become suddenly active and turned it into a virulent poison". A public analyst and adviser to the Bundaberg City Council, Jacob Christensen, condemned the purchase of the serum in bulk instead of in single dose ampoules. He said that when the rubber cap of a multiple dose bottle was pierced it was possible for a hole to be left through which air could pass carrying enormous quantities of foreign bacteria. He added "We have economised by buying serum in bulk but we have spent dearly in precious lives". One report said that the parents had all expressed their personal sympathy with Dr Thomson assuring him they had no fault to find with his work. A week later, the *Truth* commented:

> Did Dr Thomson make, even unwittingly, an error which might have contributed to the turning of the serum into a virulent toxin while it was in his possession. . .
>
> No suggestion can be entertained against Dr Thomson's conscientiousness and integrity or against any other person but the Commission must recognise, as no doubt Dr Thomson, himself, recognises that no human being ever born is beyond the range of grievous error — if an error really has been made — sometime in his career. Again, the result of the enquiry may prove that the trouble was caused by an hitherto unknown scientific reaction.
>
> The natural distress of the doctor is shared to some extent by some of his friends and at least four of the bereaved parents have called on him, deep in their sorrow as they are, to bid him well and to assure him that even the death of their own beloved kiddies has not marred their confidence in him.
>
> People speaking of him in Bundaberg as a man among medical men and it is told that he has travelled miles at times to succour some impoverished family with never any thought of ever sending them a bill.

Early in its investigations the commission learnt that for technical reasons, antiseptic, which was usually included in diphtheria serum, was omitted from the batch from which the Bundaberg bottle was drawn. There was no indication on the label or in accompanying literature of the absence of antiseptic. Analysis revealed that the remainder of the fluid in the bottle contained an organism of the staphylococcal group, which produces pus. This organism was not found in any of the bottles from the same batch recalled from many parts of Australia. When the germ was introduced into diphtheria serum containing antiseptic it failed to grow but it multiplied if the serum contained no antiseptic. Dr Thomson cooperated with the commission in every way and willingly demonstrated the technique he had used to draw up the serum and give the injections. The commission found that by picking the needles out of sterile water in which he had placed them after sterilizing them with spirit he could have contaminated both the water and the remaining needles. Experiments revealed that under certain circumstances serum without antiseptic could be contaminated from the air.

In its report published on 13 June 1928, the commission gave its opinion that the injections of toxin-antitoxin administered by Dr Thomson on 27 January 1928 were responsible for the deaths and that the immediate cause of the fatalities was the injection of live staphylococcal germs. While not ruling out the possibility of the serum being infected from the air the commission believed it had been contaminated by the doctor. The germs found in the remaining fluid were not usually found in air. The report condemned the issue of serum without antiseptic when it was intended for use on more than one occasion and advocated post-graduate training in immunization techniques. The Brisbane daily press printed large extracts of the commission's report and devoted editorials to its conclusions. The *Telegraph* stated that events had shown that there were avoidable elements in the treatment of these particular children, which removed all suspicion from the method of immunization for prevention of diphtheria but revealed the need for more stringent conditions for its practice. This paper highlighted the section of the report condemning the absence of antiseptic from the serum. The *Brisbane Courier* did not accept the commission's opinion that the serum had most probably been contaminated by Dr Thomson's technique and claimed that the evidence in this regard was not clear. It seemed satisfied with the commission's statement that immunization was the only specific measure known for the control of the disease and believed that the children must be protected.

Shortly after the publication of the Royal Commission's report, the Commonwealth Government announced that it would pay £100 to the parent or guardian of each child who had died as a result of the Bundaberg serum tragedy and also pay the whole of the medical, nursing and other incidental expenses of the children who had been inoculated but who had recovered. The announcement containing the following ambiguous statement: "The Government desires it to be clearly understood that there was no suggestion that the amount was compensation as no compensation could adequately mend these sad cases. It was a natural assumption of an obligation which was right and proper in the circumstances should be assumed by the Government." Was this an admission that the government was accepting blame for the absence of antiseptic in the Bundaberg serum which had been made by the Commonwealth Serum Laboratories?

While the authorities and the press were in favour of immunization campaigns recommencing there was some hesitation on the part of parents to allow their children to receive the injections. Gradually the local authorities took the advice that, properly administered, there would be no harmful effects, and started new programmes. The response built up over the years and soon reports came in that over ninety per cent of children commencing school in Queensland had been immunized. In Bundaberg, however, a prejudice against the procedure remained. The council began offering immunization again in 1934, six years after the tragedy. The response was below the rest of Queensland for many years.

This reluctance of the Bundaberg parents to accept the assurances that no harm would come to their children by such measures was reflected in their response to the state's offer of vaccination against poliomyelitis in 1956. In the months leading to this new campaign an accident occurred in America not unlike the Bundaberg tragedy. The Salk vaccine, used in the early years of poliomyelitis protection, was made by killing the polio virus with formaldehyde. One batch of the vaccine in which all the polio virus had not been killed resulted in the deaths of several children from poliomyelitis instead of protection against the disease. The Queensland press gave the story extensive coverage but when the consent forms were issued for the vaccination the response was excellent. Apparently parents were satisfied that the precautions by the Commonwealth Serum Laboratories and an independent testing laboratory would ensure that the Australian vaccine would be safe. Throughout the State over ninety per cent of parents consented to have their children receive the Salk vaccine. There was one exception — Bundaberg. In that city there was still a fear in some parents' minds that there would be a repetition of what happened when the diphtheria campaign commenced twenty-eight years before, and the response was less than eighty per cent. The *Bundaberg News–Mail* and radio 4BU assured the people that the vaccine to be used was perfectly safe and the technique to be used could not possibly result in any infection. The parents who had doubts were not impressed. The paper published an account of the sons of the Queensland premier, Vincent Gair, and of the director general of health and medical services, Abraham Fryberg, receiving injections from an advance supply of the vaccine. There was no improvement in response. Then Abraham Fryberg decided to enlist the help of Edward Walsh, the deputy-premier and member for Bundaberg, with whom he was friendly. Not long before the vaccination campaign was due to commence a photograph appeared on the front page of the *Bundaberg News–Mail.* It pictured young David Walsh, the grandson of the deputy-premier, sitting on his grandfather's knee receiving an injection of Salk vaccine. Within the next week the response rate in Bundaberg reached the state level.

Fraud or Medical Genius

> My mother thought she was wonderful. My father said that she was a quack. She gave my brother two grains of Condy's Crystals a day for his infantile rheumatism. All it did was turn him brown.

Thus did a Darling Downs resident describe Elizabeth Kenny, whose unorthodox treatment for infantile paralysis was the subject of a heated controversy in the 1930s and 1940s. When the disease first appeared it attacked mainly young children. As time passed, the sufferers included many in the older age groups and the name used was generally poliomyelitis. The controversy raged at a time when vaccination for the disease was still a long way off and news of a case instilled terror in the hearts of parents. Many sufferers died and more were left hopeless cripples. At first Elizabeth Kenny was ridiculed, then bitterly attacked as a quack and finally ignored by most of the Queensland medical profession. However, six Brisbane doctors who believed that her methods achieved better results than orthodox treatment, gave her a letter of introduction to colleagues in America. In that country, the Kenny method was widely accepted and she became a national heroine.

Elizabeth Kenny was born at Warialda, New South Wales, on 20 September 1880. Her father, Michael Kenny, was an Irish immigrant who had taken up a selection there. Her mother, Mary Moore, was the daughter of an Irish father and an English mother. Michael Kenny had restless feet so the family moved several times. They came to Headington Hill on the Darling Downs, Queensland, when Elizabeth was twelve and finally settled near Nobby. These frequent changes resulted in limited education for the girl at small primary schools. When she was thirteen, Elizabeth broke her wrist in a fall from a horse. Her parents drove her in a horse and buggy thirty miles to Toowoomba to attend Aeneas McDonnell, a rising surgeon and later doyen of the medical profession on the Darling Downs. McDonnell insisted young Elizabeth stay in his house while the fracture mended. Returning to her home she grew into a good-looking, strapping young woman. Her younger brother Willie, unlike

Elizabeth, was a puny child. Liza, as the family called her, worried about Willie's poor physique. In Toowoomba on one occasion, she consulted her friend Aeneas McDonnell about the problem. He suggested a series of exercises for the boy and lent Elizabeth a book on anatomy. Under his sister's supervision, Willie carried out daily exercises on a home-made machine. After months of this regime, the lad developed a fine stature.

When she was twenty-seven Elizabeth went to stay with her ageing grandmother at Guyra, and worked as a volunteer in a small maternity hospital. Despite later claims, this was the only training Elizabeth Kenny underwent as a nurse, a fact confirmed by the New South Wales and the Queensland nurses registration boards. Often she stayed in the homes of mothers experiencing problems after the birth of their babies. Elizabeth returned to her home on the Darling Downs, taking a nurse's uniform and cap made for her by a Guyra tailor.

She now set herself up as a self-appointed home nurse, riding on horseback from the farmhouse and giving her services free of charge to any who called her. Grateful patients often came later to her home bringing farm produce, poultry and cakes in return. On a summer day in 1911, she was seen riding in haste to the farm of a young couple with a two-year-old daughter. On arrival, the bush nurse was presented with something she had not seen before. The feverish little girl lay crying in her cot unable to move her legs and one arm. Puzzled by the case, Elizabeth rode several miles to the nearest telegraph station to send a message to her friend Aeneas McDonnell in Toowoomba. Some hours later back came the disturbing reply: "Infantile Paralysis — No known treatment — Do the best you can with the symptoms presenting — Aeneas J. McDonnell." Returning to the sick girl, Elizabeth tried various home-made poultices without relief. Then she tore a blanket into strips, and soaked the pieces in hot water. Wringing them out, she wrapped them around the little patient's limbs as foments. The pain eased and the little girl fell asleep. In a day or so, the nurse began passive movements of the limbs and encouraged the child to try to move them herself. Any medical man of the period would have been horrified. The traditional treatment for infantile paralysis was to immobilize the affected parts with splints. The same treatment was used on five other children in the district suffering from the disease with varying degrees of paralysis. Some months later, when Dr McDonnell enquired of the severity of the paralysis, he was surprised to hear that all of them had recovered completely. Spontaneous recovery occurs in the disease in some cases. Complete recovery in six severe cases, as he believed they had been, was rare.

Not long after this, Elizabeth Kenny opened a cottage hospital in Clifton to treat any type of case. Under the 1911 health act, local authorities had been given the power to register private hospitals. It is not known whether St Canice's Hospital, as Elizabeth had called it, was ever registered. It is certain that had she applied to the Clifton Shire Council approval would have been granted. Considering the distance from other institutions in the days of slow travel, and the service it would have given the community, the absence of formal nurse training would have been no hindrance to such approval.

Then came World War I. Elizabeth Kenny wanted to play her part for her country. She could produce no evidence of nurse registration to join the nursing service. However, taking with her a letter from Aeneas McDonnell about her work, she set off for the recruiting office. The letter from Dr McDonnell was accepted as sufficient proof of nursing experience and soon she was Staff-nurse Kenny of the Australian Army Nursing Service. She spent most of her four years war service on ships bringing back the wounded to Australia. In November 1917, she was promoted to Sister and she used this title for the rest of her life.

On returning home to Nobby she found that the district had been struck by a severe influenza epidemic that was raging throughout the world. One of her first tasks was nursing the sufferers in makeshift wards in the Clifton showgrounds. The epidemic over, she resumed her home nursing. Then came a special call from Guyra. Daphne Cregan, the seven-year-old daughter of a young woman whom Elizabeth had helped to dress for her wedding, was a spastic cripple, unable to walk. Could Elizabeth do anything to help? The unfortunate girl was brought to the farmhouse at Nobby. After many months of hot baths, passive exercises and encouragement to move her limbs herself, Daphne could manage a clumsy gait. On returning to Guyra with the much improved girl, a young doctor was so enthusiastic with the results that she suggested to Elizabeth that she demonstrate her methods to Professor Hunter, professor of Anatomy at the University of Sydney. Unfortunately Hunter died and nothing more came of the suggestion. But a germ of an idea had been planted in Elizabeth Kenny's head. She had something that she could teach the doctors.

In 1926, in a daring move for a forty-six-year-old single woman, Elizabeth Kenny adopted a ten-year-old Brisbane girl, Mary Stewart. Red-headed Mary spent her teenage years in Nobby and grew into a sweet-natured young country woman. Always interested in women's affairs, Elizabeth Kenny became the first president of the Nobby branch of the Queensland Country Women's Association.

In 1926, she also invented the "Sylvia" stretcher. A little girl had met with an accident while riding a plough, and Elizabeth was horrified at the way it was intended to transport the victim to Toowoomba. So she improvised a stretcher to make her journey more comfortable. She then set about designing a stretcher, named the Sylvia after the little girl, that would reduce shock in the transport of accident cases. It was patented and sold in many countries.

In 1930, Elizabeth Kenny answered another request to provide individual treatment for a cripple. Using similar methods to those she had used to help spastic Daphne Cregan to walk, she achieved the same results with Maude Rollenson, who had suffered from infantile paralysis eight years previously. Working with Kenny on a station property at Homestead, west of Townsville, the girl was able to hobble slowly for the first time since her illness. Then from Townsville came first one, then more requests for help. In that city in 1932 she established herself in a backyard clinic, treating seventeen patients who were spastic or long-term poliomyelitis cases. Now fifty-two years of age, Sister Kenny was in fact just beginning her real career. Splints, braces and calipers were discarded; salt baths and foments given; passive exercises conducted and active movements encouraged. Her results so impressed some of Townsville's medical practitioners, including Henry Taylor, Vennard O'Neill and Rae Dungan, that a letter was written to the state health department. As a result, arrangements were made for Sister Kenny to demonstrate her methods in Brisbane and thus began a bitter controversy which lasted several years. A strong-willed Kenny with a fanatical belief in her ability was generally opposed by a conservative medical profession, adhering to traditional treatment. At a demonstration before Aubrey Pye, medical superintendent of the Brisbane Hospital, Harold Crawford, orthopaedic specialist and president of the Queensland Branch of the Australasian Massage Association (later changed to the Physiotherapy Association), doctors, and members of the massage staff of the hospital, Sister Kenny advocated the discarding of splints and other forms of immobilization, and early active movement. One doctor said the method was criminal and Kenny's rather clumsy attempts to explain her theory of how the disbilities were caused in poliomyelitis were ridiculed.

The meeting broke up in disarray. The kindly Aubrey Pye took Sister Kenny to supper at his residence. He related afterwards that Elizabeth Kenny told him and his wife that she possessed a God-given gift to treat the disease.

Despite the unhappy outcome of her demonstration in Brisbane, Sister Kenny continued her work in Townsville where she still had the support of parents and the public. A further approach to the Queensland government was made through northern cabinet ministers, Maurice Hynes and John Dash. Ned Hanlon, the home secretary, arranged for Dr Raphael Cilento, then with the commonwealth health department, to report on the Kenny method. In December 1933, Cilento reported that Sister Kenny had produced results that inspired confidence in both lay and medical witnesses, and in several cases, these results had been achieved on patients that medical men had stated would no further respond to the orthodox methods. He added that Sister Kenny might be achieving her results by suggestion or perhaps by some special facility of touch that she possessed. Cilento recommended that the Queensland government provide funds for a clinic in which the progress of her patients might be observed and a judgment made on her ability to teach her method to others.

Darling Downs polio nurse Elizabeth Kenny demonstrated her revolutionary techniques for combating the paralysis of polio in 1940. (Courtesy Queensland Department of Health)

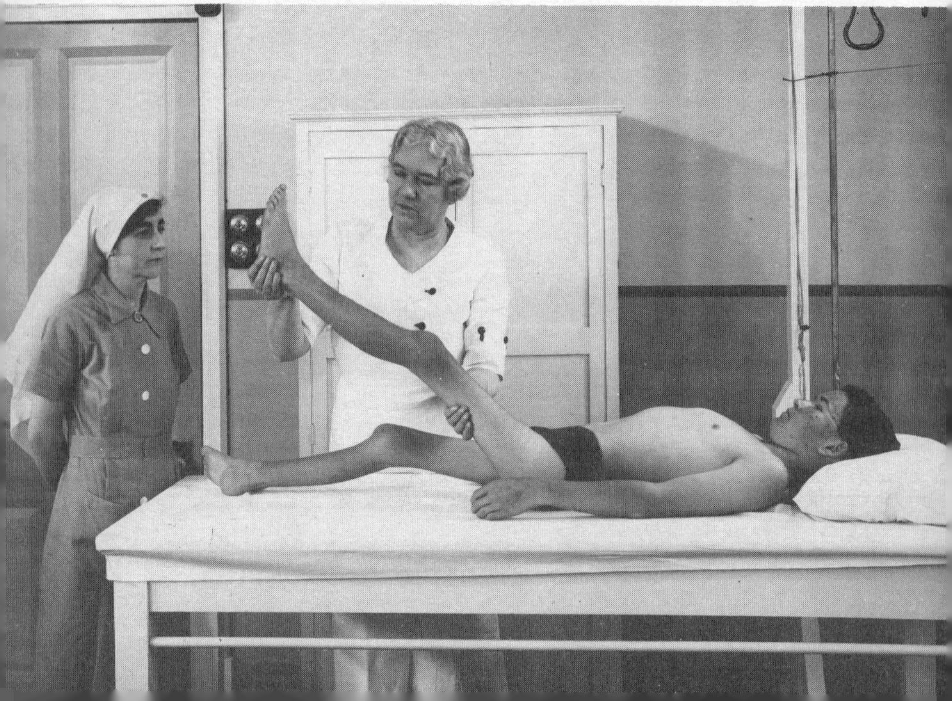

Accordingly, a clinic was established in the Queen's Hotel, Townsville. The son of the proprietress of the hotel was a young doctor, James Guinane, then overseas. On his return, he became involved in the clinic and was at times over-enthusiastic, making exaggerated claims for the results obtained. Cilento reported again six months later. He stated that there had been a general improvement in all cases studied but the great majority of the patients were cases whose treatment had previously been neglected. He added that in training others, the clinic had failed as the nurses had not acquired the necessary proficiency to conduct the treatment on their own.

After the criticism and the ridicule she had received previously in Brisbane, Sister Kenny had not retaliated. However this time she reacted immediately, as she was to do in the future whenever she was criticized. She wrote a long reply to Hanlon, the home secretary, disputing Cilento's report. Hanlon went to Townsville himself and was so impressed with what he saw that he arranged for a clinic to be established in Brisbane at the corner of George and Charlotte streets. Sister Kenny came down from Townsville to supervise treatment, and Jean Rountree was appointed medical superintendent, a position later occupied by Abe Fryberg. The new clinic received great publicity and requests for treatment were received not only from Queensland but from other parts of Australia and overseas. Further clinics were established at Cairns, Rockhampton and Toowoomba in Queensland, North Shore Hospital and Newcastle in New South Wales, and in Melbourne.

There was still bitter opposition from many doctors. James Duhig, a prominent pathologist in Brisbane, wrote: "this quack must be exposed". In April 1935, Cilento, now director general of health and medical services in the state Health department, and knighted in the previous New Year's honours list, made a press statement in which he advocated more funds for the orthodox treatment instead of financing the "more spectacular endeavour" of the Kenny clinics. He was strangely offside with the official opinion of his own department, espoused by Hanlon and by Chuter, the assistant undersecretary who was an ardent supporter of Sister Kenny throughout her career. Despite the general medical opposition, parents and the public strongly supported Elizabeth Kenny. In October 1936, the citizens of Townsville gave her a civic reception in the Theatre Royal. The mayor of Townsville, Alderman J.S.M. Gill, said that "as the public of Townsville have recognized the splendid courage and skill of this noble woman, so did they demonstrate their appreciation on the first occasion on which they have had an opportunity of expressing their admiration for her and her gift to humanity". Later, a playground in the city was dedicated in her honour.

In October 1935, the government appointed a royal commission of Queensland doctors to enquire into the treatment of infantile paralysis generally and the Kenny method in particular. The first members were C.A. Thelander, chairman, A.J. McDonnell, L.J. Nye, J. Bostock, J.R.S. Lahz, A.E. Paterson and J.V. Duhig, with Jean Rountree as liaison officer. Later, Dr L. Gibson joined the commission and Dr Bostock resigned. It was to be more than two years before the commission reported. In the meantime not all doctors were opposed to the Kenny method. Herbert Wilkinson, professor of Anatomy at the new Queensland Medical School, supported her and wrote a foreword to a book she published in 1937, entitled, *Infantile Paralysis and Cerebral Diplegia*. In the same year, grateful parents of a spastic patient paid her fare to England, and she was given two wards at Queen Mary's Hospital, at Carshalton. She shocked English doctors with her blunt condemnation of the orthodox treatment they had been using and her recommendation to discard splinting and commence active movement in the early stages of the disease. Returning to Australia in 1938, she was greeted with the report of the Queensland royal commission. It damned her methods, stating that "the abandonment of immobilization is a grievous error and fraught with great danger, especially in very young children who cannot cooperate in reeducation". It added that it "could not recommend the application of the Kenny method of treatment of cripples at any stage of paralysis and especially not in the treatment of the acute or early stage". The *Courier-Mail* reported Cilento commenting that "Sister Kenny had considerably watered down her claims. She no longer insisted as she did in 1934 that she began where doctors left off. . . It was gratifying to him to know that in each case the reports entirely confirmed the points he made in his independent report of 1934."

Despite this setback, the Queensland government still supported her, even to the extent of giving her a ward at the Brisbane Hospital. For the first time she was able to treat cases in the early stage of the disease. Some of her therapists worked in the infectious block applying hot packs and giving early active movement to patients whose parents had chosen the Kenny method. When the infectious stage was over, these patients were transferred to her ward. Aubrey Pye, the superintendent, had this to say of her treatment.

> Her patients recovered more quickly. Their limbs were more supple and much better nourished. Sister Kenny was given all the trained nurses she required. She taught them her methods of treatment. All day they had no other duties or patients to nurse. Kenny often spent much of the night with her patients depending on their condition. The hospital patients were seen perhaps three times a week by the visiting medical officer, each day by a senior resident medical officer and maybe not more than once by the physiotherapist depending on their condition. She well demonstrated the value of intensive care and treatment. She sought as much contact with the medical profession as possible but she was almost completely ignored. The medical profession was invited to accompany her on rounds of her patients in ward 7. In this ward there was a marked contrast between the patients she had treated from the outset of the illness and those she had not. It must be appreciated that this was in the war years. Because of the large number of medical officers in the services those left in civilian practice and on the hospital staff were exceptionally busy. Only the odd practitioner other than the resident medical officers I could round up bothered to attend. Sometimes Dr Jarvis Nye and Alan Lee came. It was interesting how quickly she could catch on to an idea or comment. On the next round she might have incorporated it in her treatment as if it were her idea.

With this widespread apathy among the Queensland medical profession, six Brisbane doctors who did support her — Arden, Fryberg, Lee, Nye, Pye and Wilkinson — suggested she go to America. An approach was made to the government and the idea was supported. The premier, Forgan Smith, wrote to Basil O'Connor, president of the American National Foundation for Infantile Paralysis. He said that "in the opinion of the Queensland Government and that of medical men, Miss Kenny has made a notable contribution to the cause of humanity. Miss Kenny has given her services entirely voluntarily and has neither sought nor accepted any monetary reward from the Government or from patients". The home secretary, Hanlon, at a farewell function, presented Sister Kenny with a cheque to cover fares for herself and her ward Mary Stewart-Kenny who had been trained as a therapist. Her medical supporters provided a letter of introduction to the famous Mayo Clinic.

Arriving in America in 1940, her reception was at first disheartening. Basil O'Connor was absent from New York; Morris Fishbein, editor of the journal of the American Medical

Association in Chicago, thought she was a crank and the doctors at the Mayo Clinic were polite but did not treat poliomyelitis cases. However, the clinic doctors gave her a letter of introduction to doctors at nearby Minneapolis where there were plenty of polio cases. Again, most doctors rejected the interpretation of the terms of "spasm", "mental alienation" and "incoordination" she used to explain her theories of how the disabilities were caused when a patient contracted poliomyelitis. However, there were three exceptions. They were orthopaedic specialists Miland Knapp, John Pohl and Wallace Cole. After demonstrating her methods on individual cases she was given beds in the Minneapolis General Hospital. Her three sponsors were pleased with her results. In June 1941, the American Medical Association published a preliminary report of the Kenny method by Cole and Knapp. They said that "the patients were much more comfortable and cheerful during the acute stage than those who are immobilized. Certainly harm has not resulted to any of the observed patients under Sister Kenny's care from the abandonment of immobilization". Not long after the preliminary report, the National Foundation of Infantile Paralysis also reported favourably. Then in December 1941, the treatment was stamped with the imprimatur of the American Medical Association in an editorial in its journal. After being damned by the Queensland royal commission three years before, her use of heat for spasm and pain, no immobilization and early movement were now widely accepted by the American doctors. She began courses for doctors and physiotherapists from the rest of America and from many parts of the world. The Sister Kenny Institute was established in Minneapolis in 1942 and other Kenny clinics were opened. She accepted numerous invitations to lecture in other countries and received honorary degrees from three universities — Rutgers, New York and Rochester. Becoming a national heroine, she required police assistance at one New York function as the crowd slashed buttons from her frock and tried to souvenir her hat. For several years, the American public placed her second to Eleanor Roosevelt, the wife of the American president, in a poll to name the most admired woman. Her autobiography, written in collaboration with Martha Ostenso, was published under the title *And They Shall Walk*. In 1946, Elizabeth Kenny was eulogized in the film, *Sister Kenny* in which Rosalind Russell played the key role. Four years later the American Congress by special act granted her the rare honour of free access to the United States without any formalities. Such an honour had been granted only twice before — to La Fayette and Winston Churchill.

Despite these successes, however, there was often bitter controversy, partly due to the attitude of those who still opposed her, and partly due to her own personality. Not known for her graciousness, her criticism of opponents was generally merciless and became more so as time went on. There were no half measures. She wanted total acceptance of her methods by all the medical profession. Those who modified her approach often suffered the same tongue lashing as those who rejected her method entirely. Even the Kenny Institute in Minneapolis did not escape her criticism, which the staff found tiresome.

Elizabeth Kenny was not without humour. A large woman, with grey and later white hair which she covered with large hats, she was a noticeable figure. She often told the tale of how when walking George Street, Brisbane, one day, she heard a little boy cry, "Hey, Mum! There goes Mae West." In 1946, the Queensland government sent Abe Fryberg, then deputy director general of health and medical services, and Tom Stubbs Brown, orthopaedic specialist, overseas to study the latest treatment of poliomyelitis, including the current position of the Kenny method. Getting out of a car with Sister Kenny, the polite Stubbs Brown said, "Sister Kenny, would you trust me with your papers?" To which she replied, "Dr Brown, I would trust you with anything except a case of poliomyelitis." This jibe was not held against her — when the two investigators submitted their report it upheld her treatment for the early stages of the disease. However they stated that her concept that the disabilities were caused by the virus invading the peripheral tissues and not the central nervous system, as traditionally held, was not proven.

She returned to Australia several times during her American career, generally without acclaim. In the *Courier-Mail* Harry Summers wrote that "merits or demerits of her treatment apart, it is a real achievement to have come out of a Queensland bush town and become a world figure. The only women's organization to give her a public welcome was the Toowoomba branch of the Country Women's Association. Charles Chuter, the official responsible for her first reception by the government, was as faithful as ever to her cause".

But Sister Kenny developed Parkinson's Disease, and retired to Toowoomba in 1951. The last months saw her writing a book — published posthumously — *My Battle and Victory*. She also involved herself in an organization called The International

Organisation for Combating Poliomyelitis. She died on 30 November 1952. The service in the Neil Street Methodist Church was broadcast throughout the world by the Australian Broadcasting Commission, and she was buried in the Nobby cemetery. The Toowoomba citizens erected a memorial sundial at the entrance to the public baths. In Nobby stands a modest memorial erected by the local branch of the Country Women's Association. In 1981, the government named a recently acquired building that stands where the Brisbane Kenny Clinic was located, Kenny House. H.J. Seddon, noted British orthopaedist wrote the following in an obituary in the British Medical Journal:

> The influence of Sister Kenny on the treatment of infantile paralysis has been exceedingly beneficial. One of the great misconceptions that gave rise to an immense amount of crippling was that strict immobilisation was thought to be necessary in the early days of the disease. Sister Kenny went to the other extreme, and perhaps too far, in abandoning practically all forms of splinting; but she was undoubtedly on the right lines, and surgeons in many countries who have been influenced by her ideas in this respect are finding their patients have much less muscle wasting and joint stiffness than formerly.
>
> Sister Kenny was a woman with a mission, and she was so convinced she was right that she attacked all her critics mercilessly. It was useless to point out that her ideas of the treatment of poliomyelitis changed fairly rapidly as increasing contact with able medical people and other physiotherapists added to her initial small store of knowledge. But in an empirical way she hit on much that is good in the treatment of poliomyelitis, and her vigour was such that she wakened orthopaedic surgeons and physiotherapists the world over. Had she been content to talk about treatment without speculations about pathology, and had she been a little kindlier and more tolerant, she might now be regarded as the Florence Nightingale of orthopaedics, or at any rate of that part of it concerned with poliomyelitis.

Her biographer, Victor Cohn, asked this question: "How can we explain this woman who was called both a fraud and a medical genius, a cheap quack and an unhappy martyr, a raging old tiger and a merciful angel?"

A Short Funeral

One of the most colourful personalities to enter the Queensland parliament was Tom Aikens, independent member for Mundingburra and later Townsville South, for over thirty years. In 1960, author Clem Lack summed him up:

> Mr Aikens is a dyed in the wool Independent, although he denies the label. He is the most forthright and truculent independent Independent to enter Parliament in the last 25 years — a political buccaneer who trains his guns impartially on the Government and Opposition benches and neither gives nor asks for quarter. He is one of the ablest and certainly the most unorthodox of debaters. A gifted singer, he has an excellent voice which can be measured in decibels when he desires to be heard by Mr Speaker above a roar of hostile interjectors. A frank and unblushing egotist, Mr Aikens has a gift of vivid and unexpected phrase which he can use like a cutlass to cut down an opponent or as a rapier in a verbal thrust and parry.

In 1969, the minister for health, S.D. (later Sir Douglas) Tooth, introduced a bill to amend the Medical Act. The bill covered postmortems, organ transplants and the legibility of doctor's handwriting. Tom Aikens's speech on the bill can be found in the *Queensland Parliamentary Debates*:

> MR AIKENS: (Townsville South) (12.46 p.m.): When I was listening to the Minister's introduction of this measure I gathered the impression that the purpose of the Bill was purely and simply to clarify certain legal points which had arisen, and that action is, of course, always desirable. Far too often now does that have to be done, and I hope that one of these days Ministers will introduce Bills that are so clear and unambiguous that they can be read and interpreted by anybody.
>
> I also gained the impression that this Bill, like most Bills introduced in this Chamber, was drawn up by "city slickers" with no knowledge of what goes on outside the perimeter of Brisbane. I do not say that in a derogatory sense, and certainly not derisively. It is quite true that over the years doctors have got into the habit of writing indecipherable certificates and prescriptions. Indeed, it seems to be almost a status symbol with some of them. I know some doctors who can write very clearly and very well but who, when called upon to

write a certificate or a prescription, write in such a way that only a chemist can understand. I am reminded of the story of the young girl who took a love letter to a chemist in Townsville and said to him, "Will you please read this for me? My sweetheart is a doctor." Perhaps it is just as well sometimes that patients cannot read what doctors write.

We know, of course, that there is academic Latin, and there is also "dog" Latin, as used by the medical profession. As a keen student of languages and, as a matter of fact, a rather outstanding linguist, I know something of these things. One day a fellow brought a doctor's prescription to me and said, "I must be pretty crook. Look at all the stuff written on this prescription." With my knowledge of "dog" Latin I interpreted it for him that the doctor had written on it for the chemist, "I have had my cut out of this guy. Now it's your turn." He took the prescription to a chemist who gave him some coloured water and charged him an exhorbitant price. These days, when representatives of pharmaceutical firms walk into chemist shops all day with tablets, potions and pills, I wonder how many chemists could really interpret an old-style doctor's prescription, with all the various medicaments that had to be measured and mixed in a certain way.

I now want to be more serious and deal with post-mortem examinations. Let us remember that the doctor who opens the cadaver takes from it certain organs, snippings from other organs and samples of liquids and so on from various parts of the body and sends them away to various institutes for examination. If a post-mortem certificate is required, sometimes it is necessary, even in a large provincial city, to wait a fortnight. This is not because the doctor who opened the body does not know his job but because he has to get the opinions of so many other people on what happened to the patient and what actually caused his death.

The Minister should not get the idea that the doctor who opens the cadaver is the fellow who issues the post-mortem certificate or even gives an opinion as to the cause of death. That is all very well in the capital city, provincial cities, or some of the big country towns, where there are doctors. But who is going to issue a certificate of death in the great open back country. When I lived out there, a certificate was sometimes issued by the local constable. Sometimes we could not get a constable to the dead man and we got a local J.P. to issue a certificate. If there was no J.P. we got someone to sign his name and put the letters "J.P." after it — no-one knew the difference — and we buried the dead man under the beefwood tree, or wherever we could dig a grave for him.

I will never forget an occasion when we were burying a man out in the hard schistose country that is standing on end [*sic*]. We gave two men a bottle of rum and a bag of water to go and dig the grave while we celebrated, or held a wake — hon. members can call it what they like — and then, after an appropriate time, we put the corpse into a coffin made out of an old piano case, put it into a spring-cart drawn by an old grey horse and drove to the place where the man was to be buried. When we got there, we found the two gravediggers in the shade of a tree well under the weather, with the grave about 4 ft. 6 ins. long and only 3 feet deep. We had an itinerant parson with us, and we tried to put the coffin into the grave this way, that way, and some other way, but we could not get it in. We did not know what we could do to solve the problem, but one man said, "Leave it to me." He unhooked the old grey horse from the spring-cart, threw the traces over its back, trotted back to the shanty, and came back with a cross-cut saw. We cut through the coffin and severed the fellow's legs just below the knees — we measured the grave first — and put him in that way, and he went to his reward just as well as if he had been buried by one of the leading ecclesiastics of the country. That man obviously was dead, and he was buried. We all knew what he had died from. He had been crawling through a wire fence with a double-barrelled shotgun and was foolish enough to crawl through first and pull the shotgun after him, instead of pushing the shotgun through first and crawling through afterwards, and he shot himself. We all knew what had happened to him.

What is going to happen in the back country when no doctor is available to perform a post-mortem and it is not possible to bring a doctor in to perform one? Even in these days of the aerial ambulance, there are times when it cannot land because of boggy conditions or other adverse conditions. In some instances the corpse is so decomposed that it is very difficult to ascertain what caused the death; but the man is obviously dead and he has to be buried — unless one leaves him there for the goannas to eat. It is all very well to write into this legislation clauses that obviously are capable of implementing in the capital city, the provincial cities, and the big country towns, but are worthless out in the back country.

Even when a patient dies in a big country town there is sometimes a dispute as to the cause of death. I remember a famous murder case in Charters Towers some years ago in which a woman was found dead in the heart of the town. About a fortnight or so after she had died a man was arrested and charged with her murder. He should have gone to gaol for life; there was no doubt that he had murdered her, but the doctors of Charters Towers could not ascertain the cause of death. The various organs and snippings were sent down to pathologists and other departmental experts in Brisbane, but they could not pin-point the cause of death. So, because there was no actual evidence from any competent doctor as to the cause of the woman's death, the murderer went free — and I have not the slightest hesitation in branding him a murderer. If the woman's body had been found, say, a day or two after death, the doctors could have pin-pointed the cause of death and that man would have gone to gaol; he would have been convicted of murder.

After a body lies some time and decomposition takes place, and certain other elements come into focus, as it were, there is no possible chance of any doctor in certain cases, pin-pointing the cause of death. Let us face up to these things. With regard to heart transplantations, ever since I first heard about them I have considered them as purely and simply surgical showmanship. I think it will be many years — perhaps never — a body can completely absorb a new heart. Any surgeon who has done other medical transplantation work, such as corneas and various other things, knows the difficulties involved. I feel sure the hon. member for Wavell (Dr Crawford) — no-one would know better than he — was envisaging difficulties when he asked the Minister to-day a question with regard to the equipment required for renal transplantation. I know it has been done successfully and it is a wonderful thing. Very shortly, I suppose, doctors will be transplanting other organs into the human body and I think it is very wise that we should have at least the consent of the —

Mr Lickiss interjected.

Mr AIKENS: I suggest to the hon. member that a head transplant would not be a bad idea. Even if the donor of it was the hon. member for Rockhampton North it would be an improvement.

Mr Porter: Do you know everything?

MR AIKENS: No, I do not know everything, but at least I try to learn. The real boss of my political organisation has never rushed into the Press and said that something I said in this House is prattling. I have never been accused of prattling by any body.

Mr W.D. Hewitt interjected.

MR AIKENS: Oh, the Hewitt histrionics, The Chinchen casuistry, the Murray mumblings and the Lickess licence. That alliteration —

The CHAIRMAN: Order!

MR AIKENS: Let us face to every Bill before this Chamber and all other business that comes before us with the knowledge we have of it. None of us can say that we know everything of it. Let every one of us go out, as I always do, as a simple seeker after truth and not as one who professes to know everything as so many members of this Chamber do.

I really believe that we should wait quite a long time before we permit heart transplants in this country. With regard to other organ transplants, it is necessary to get the permission of the donor himself before he dies or his nearest surviving relative. But there again a legal point can be raised and the Minister might ask the legal officers to have a look at it. Do hon. members know that if someone provides in his will that his body be given to the university, or that one of his organs be given to somewhere else — to some school of anatomy for transplanting — or makes provision for cremation or that no burial service be performed by a minister of religion, that is not binding on anybody? Do hon. members know that the executors of their wills, if they do not want to, in law need not carry out their wishes, that what they write in their wills is merely their own wish and is not binding on anybody? I think only the actual disposition of their assets is binding on their executors.

Mr Ramsden: It is binding unless the next of kin agrees otherwise.

MR AIKENS: It is not binding at all unless the executor wishes to comply with it.

The CHAIRMAN: Order!

MR AIKENS: That is referred to in the legal phrase, "Your beneficiary agrees to opt".

Mr Murray: We will check with Col Bennet.

MR AIKENS: If we bring the hon. member for South Brisbane into it we will probably be in a worse fog than ever.

(Sitting suspended from 1 to 2.15 p.m.)

MR AIKENS: I had said that there was a need for the Minister to clean up certain legal aspects in regard to people who bequeath their bodies to medical schools for dissection or will parts of their bodies or organs for transplant purposes. We should face up to the fact that many people, like myself, do not care very much what happens to their bodies or any part of their bodies after death. In my own family there is some little disputation at the present time because very strong representations are being made from abroad to have me buried in Westmister Abbey, with the rest of the Empire's most illustrious dead, whereas it is a matter of complete indifference to me whether or not I am cut up and used for cray-bait.

If I remember rightly, some time ago a Bill was passed to give the Minister power to order a blood transfusion where a blood transfusion was considered necessary to save the life of a patient. In these days of what are termed ratbag religious organisations, we know that some parents will not give their consent to their children having blood transfusions even when the transfusions will save the children's lives. A Bill was introduced to vest the Minister with power to order blood transfusions where doctors consider them to be absolute necessary.

Mr W.D. Hewitt: Only for a child.

MR AIKENS: Only for a child or for a dependant.

The Bill, of course, relates to an adult who may be prevailed upon to will his body — or he may do so of his own volition — to a medical school for dissection or to bequeath certain organs of his body for transplant purposes. However, if the legal point is not cleared up it is possible that his nearest relatives may not carry out his wishes. We know that frequently and tragically families are divided on religious issues, and it is quite possible that a wife may be divided from her husband on the matter of religion. She may be the main beneficiary in her husband's will and, under our law, as it was explained to me, can object even to the terms of the will.

In my will I have made provision — and it is still there — for my body to be cremated and I have stipulated that there shall be no funeral service of any religious import at all delivered by anyone connected with any religious organization. I have said that there should be no flowers or headstone on my grave in the event of my not being cremated. When I made my will the man who drafted it for me — he later became a top-ranking legal officer in this State — said, "Tom, I hope you will remember that all those things with regard to the disposal of your body and burial are merely requests and that if your family does not consider that you should be buried in that way or if it wants some minister of religion to perform a burial service it is at liberty to have that done." Possibly the same situation might arise in regard to disposal of a man's body or parts of his body.

Mr Murray: I think that the public would want some evidence that they had at last got rid of you.

MR AIKENS: The public will know by the elation of my political enemies. As a matter of fact, the A.L.P. will throw a party lasting for three or four months, and I have no doubt that it will "take the knock" for the cost of it, the same as it "takes the knock" for some of its election expenses.

I hope that the Minister will clear up this matter and have his "legal eagles" go into to it to determine whether the relatives of a deceased person can alter the terms of his will relative to the disposal of his body or portions or organs of it. At present, as the law was explained to me by a competent man — that does not include the hon. member for South Brisbane — I know that all my requests about the disposal of my body and the funeral arrangements can be brushed aside if my family so wishes.

Mr W.D. Hewitt interjected.

MR AIKENS: To be quite candid I was thinking of leaving my body to medical science, but can the hon. members imagine what would happen to my cadaver if it were were wheeled into the room and the Liberals on this side and the Labour Party on that got busy with their axes and saws.

Mr Murray: Get Col. Bennett to draw up your will.

MR AIKENS: Let us end this levity and flippancy. We have had enough of it, although a little nonsense now and then is relished by the wisest men, as the old saying goes.

This is a serious issue and I think the best legal brains in the State should be put to work on it. I know of some people who wish to leave their bodies to the medical profession and others who wish to leave certain organs for transplant purposes. I wish to make sure that if they make a will along those lines while they are of sound mind, the terms of the will will not be upset. I point out that, in relation to the disposal of property, many people think that if they have a certain amount of money or property, they can bequeath it to whomsoever they want to.

The CHAIRMAN: Order! I hope the hon member will relate his remarks to the Bill.

MR AIKENS: I am just making this point. Anybody can have a Supreme Court Judge determine how the property of a deceased person is to be disposed of, and sometimes he decides in defiance on the terms of will. If a judge can dispose in that way of the material possessions of a deceased person — and that has been done frequently — it can be done in the case of a deceased person's body, or his organs.

The Country Needs You

When Aubrey Pye, superintendent of the Royal Brisbane Hospital from 1933 to 1967, was asked to name the changes that had taken place at the hospital during his term of office, he listed the regular supply of resident medical officers which resulted from the establishment of the Queensland Medical School as the most important. The new source of junior medical staff replaced a "catch as catch can" method of recruitment of resident medical officers from the south who joined and left the staff at whim. The first graduation from the Queensland Medical School was in 1940, but the demand on medical manpower for service in the armed forces during World War II delayed a regular supply of young doctors until after 1945. At first the Queensland graduates were absorbed mainly by the Brisbane hospitals, but as hospitals in the larger provincial cities expanded they were approved by the medical board as suitable training centres where new graduates could serve the compulsory twelve months required before full registration was granted. However, new graduates generally preferred to serve their first year after graduation at the large metropolitan hospitals with their greater facilities in most specialties. A few new doctors favoured the hospitals in the larger country centres where the junior staff were expected to accept more responsibility than in the Brisbane hospitals, but there was usually only a trickle of applicants for hospitals in the smaller country cities.

When Edward Hanlon assumed the home secretary's portfolio in 1932 and later that of Health and Home Affairs in 1935, he dreamed of a public hospital system staffed entirely by salaried medical officers. When he realized that this was not a practical proposition, he introduced central control of medical staffing by including in the 1936 Hospitals Act a provision that no hospital board could appoint a medical officer unless the director general of health and medical services approved the applicant. The legislation covered all medical staff from senior specialists to junior resident medical officers. As a result of this legislation the appointment of new graduates to their first positions in Queensland hospitals was controlled by the director general. The method of allocation depended on the grading of the graduate in his final examination and his preference of a hospital in which he hoped to spend his compulsory first year. The graduate indicated his preference by placing the hospitals in the desired order on his application form which was sent to the director general. The faculty of Medicine provided a list of successful students graded according to the total marks they had received in the final examination. When these two factors were taken as a guide in allocating the positions at Queensland hospitals, the bright students generally were appointed to hospitals of their first choice while the students at the bottom of the order of merit list received postings to hospitals well down on their preference list.

During the first decades after World War II, Queensland country hospitals experienced great difficulty obtaining medical staff owing to a universal shortage of doctors. Although hospital boards were responsible under the Hospitals Act for recruiting medical staff, they leant heavily on the director general in these difficulties. In turn, the directors general did their utmost to secure doctors for the country areas. Legend has it that when I was appointed director general in 1969, I got down on my knees each night and prayed that I would be able to recruit enough medicos for the hospitals outside the metropolitan area.

Early in 1970 I realized that staffing for 1971 would be more difficult than usual. A new award for resident medical officers had granted them reduced working hours. As a result the Health department had given approval for an additional 36 junior positions from the beginning of the new year. The difficulty was increased by a reduced number of students in the final year of 1970. Although at the beginning of their course there had been the usual number entering the first year of training, somewhere along the way an over-zealous examiner had thinned their ranks. The number of first year resident medical officer posts in Queensland was expected to be 130, with the metropolitan hospitals requiring 100 new doctors and the country hoping to recruit 30. I calculated that the Queensland Medical School would provide only 100 graduates, thus leaving 30 posts to be filled through other means. The superintendents of metropolitan hospitals came to my office to discuss the problem. The new award, while creating the difficulty, promised a solution. Salaries had been raised to a level considerably higher than that paid to resident medical officers in other states of Australia. The meeting recommended that a vigorous advertising campaign be launched to attract southern graduates to help fill the quota of first year resident medical positions in Queensland. The Health minister, Douglas Tooth, approved the recommendation and around August 1970 Queensland hospitals advertised the positions widely in all other states of Australia and New Zealand. I explained this plan to representatives of the Queensland students but as no disadvantage to Queenslanders was apparent to them, the advice was not discussed with their colleagues. A flood of applications from southern students poured into my office. At first it appeared there would be no difficulty in filling all the positions in Queensland but closer scrutiny revealed a difficulty. Most of the southern applicants were willing to serve only in Brisbane hospitals. Only a few had applied for positions outside the metropolitan area. With most Queenslanders also indicating their preference for Brisbane hospitals, I realized that there were more than enough applicants for hospitals in the capital city but only a few who were willing to serve in the 30 positions in the country. I convened another meeting with the metropolitan medical superintendents, and explained my obligation to fill the positions in the provincial city hospitals. Large Brisbane hospitals suffered little when the staff was one or two short of their quota, but the absence of one medical officer in a small country hospital placed a heavy burden on the remainder of the staff. The meeting agreed to a plan which it believed would solve the problem but would doubtless meet with great opposition.

I would use my power under the Hospitals Act to approve only seventy Queensland graduates for metropolitan hospitals. If the remainder wished to work in Queensland they would be approved for country hospitals only. The minister agreed to the proposal knowing the criticism it would bring. Southern students were advised of approval for Brisbane hospital posts on condition they passed their final examination and were willing to accept immediately. Favourable replies were received from sufficient southerners to ensure that part of the plan would be successful.

There was no attempt on the part of the Department of Health to keep the plan a secret but no official announcement was made. The first public hint was given by Arthur Crawford, a medical practitioner and the member for Wavell in the Queensland Legislative Assembly. Although a member of the Liberal Party to which the Health minister also belonged, he had attacked the Health department at every opportunity. On 12 November Crawford raised the matter in parliament. The relevant extract from Hansard reads as follows:

QUESTIONS WITHOUT NOTICE

Dr Crawford: I ask the Minister for Health: With regard to the staffing of our hospitals in the 1971 year, I understand that we will be short of medical graduates and that the Director General of Health has already announced that southern graduates will be appointed and given priority over Queensland graduates. Is this true? Does the Minister feel that by giving southern graduates the pick of the positions in Queensland, more of our own graduates will immediately migrate south, bearing in mind that 25 percent. of our honours graduates and 14 percent. of all graduates departed after graduation last year?

Mr Tooth: I have no way of knowing or even guessing, what graduates from Queensland or from the South are likely to do. However, I am very surprised that anybody in my department has stated that preference, priority or privilege will be granted to southern graduates over local graduates.

This was the beginning of several weeks of controversy in which the proposed plan of allocation was debated hotly and often emotionally, particularly by the Queensland students, hospital medical staffs and involved senior members of the profession. As director general I found that many of my acquaintances had sons or daughters among the Queensland students who might be affected by the decision. When I appeared at Parliament House to advise the minister during debates on the department's estimates or new legislation I was approached by members of the house who had relatives in the final year of medicine. Members of the council of the Australian Medical Association, well-known to me, had sons who were likely to be sent to the country under the proposed allocation. The question most often asked of me was Why couldn't all the Queensland graduates be posted to Brisbane hospitals and the southerners be sent to the country?

The controversy reached fever pitch in the last week of November. Arthur Crawford raised the matter in a detailed question. This time the minister, in a full answer, gave an explanation of the events leading up to the decision and defended the action being taken. Crawford's question and part of the minister's answer were recorded in Hansard:

Dr Crawford, pursuant to notice, asked The Minister for Health, —

Apropos of the staffing of our hospitals in 1971 and the necessity to employ southern medical graduates, matters which are of major concern to Queensland —

(1) Does he still affirm that priority is not being given to southern graduates?

(2) Have some 44 southerners, mainly Victorians, already been appointed to our major metropolitan hospitals?

(3) Does this mean that, with approximately 100 posts available to new doctors in metropolitan hospitals, only a little over half of them will then be offered to Queensland graduates whose final examination results are not yet to hand?

(4) Besides the Brisbane metropolitan posts, how many southern doctors have been appointed to country and provincial city hospitals, which are these hospitals and how many appointments were made to each?

(5) Is it considered likely that of the appointments already made to southern graduates, some may yet break their contracts to accept belated offers of positions in their home cities?

Answer:- (1 to 5) "No departure from long-established practice with respect to the allocation of first-year resident medical officers amongst approved hospitals is contemplated. There will be the usual distribution between Brisbane and the provincial cities of Queensland of graduates seeking limited registration in this State. This will be in accordance with the policy pursued hitherto which has always been designed to protect the interests of country hospitals as well as those of the metropolis. In the allocation of resident medical officers we have an obligation to try to staff country hospitals as adequately as possible. I would remind the Honourable Member for Wavell that he himself pointed out the problems and the needs of country hospitals in the debate on matters of public interest on November 18 last. To allocate all the Queensland graduates to Brisbane hospitals and none outside the metropolis would be gross discrimination against the countryside and a neglect of responsibility. . . Whilst the numbers graduating have been falling the needs of hospitals have markedly increased and it is obvious that there will be a shortage in both city and country hospitals.

In an endeavour to overcome this shortage all hospitals, both city and country, employing resident medical officers, were advised to advertise throughout Australia. The Department also advertised extensively. The response of second-year doctors was not great, only 17 applications being received and it is apparent that even with these additional applicants from other States there will be a shortage of second-year resident medical officers. The response for first-year positions was more encouraging as 90 enquiries were received. Of these seven have shown an interest in positions at Townsville, Cairns, and Toowoomba, whilst another 37 have indicated that they may accept appointments in Brisbane. Unless southern graduates are recruited there will be a shortage in both city and country.

The next day, Wednesday 26 November, Eric Saint, dean of the Queensland University faculty of Medicine, sent me the list of Queensland students who had been successful in the final examinations, arranged in order of merit. I noted that of 107 successful students, 100 had elected to serve in Queensland. But I realized that many of those at the lower end of the order of merit list whom I wished to send to country hospitals had listed only metropolitan hospitals in their preference lists. In order to appoint them in Queensland they would have to be persuaded to add the country hospitals to their application forms.

The Queensland Medical Act demanded that new graduates be granted limited registration before taking up a position in the hospital in which they were to serve their twelve months' preliminary training. In accordance with established practice the medical board had arranged that the successful 1970 Queensland students be registered as a group on Thursday 26 November at AMA House in a combined function with the Australian Medical Association which would welcome the new doctors to the profession. In the past such functions had been quite pleasant affairs. The formalities of registration were dispensed with as quickly as possible and welcoming speeches were short. Afterwards, new graduates, flushed with success, mingled with older members of the profession to receive congratulations and talk excitedly of the future. As the director general of health and medical services, I was ex officio president of the Queensland medical board. As I drove to the function I realized I would be meeting face to face a group of new doctors and older practitioners who were opposed to the plan of allocation. On arrival, I sensed a feeling of disapproval but my address, as the president of the medical board and as the director general of health, was received without any outward demonstration of hostility. I was somewhat surprised that all the graduates in the lower end of the order of merit list responded to my request to add country hospitals to their application forms. I took it as a sign that they would at least consider staying in Queensland and not depart to work elsewhere as had been suggested by the member for Wavell. However, evidence that those present at the function were doing more than exchanging congratulations and discussing future careers was revealed in the *Courier-Mail* next morning. The paper carried the following article.

PROTEST ON JOB ALLOCATION FOR NEW DOCTORS

Queensland doctors and medical students will protest against the State Health Department's decision to grant preferential appointments to southern graduates who have accepted first-year medical officer appointments in Queensland Hospitals. It is understood that the AMA will protest that Queensland graduates are not getting fair

> placement in hospitals of their own choice in their State. Already 37 southern graduates, who have missed plum appointments in their own States have contracted to serve in metropolitan hospitals. A further seven have nominated leading provincial hospitals. Many Queenslanders will miss metropolitan appointments because they have been filled from the south.

A council of the Australian Medical Association was scheduled for 8 p.m. on the day the article appeared. Key figures at the meeting were Egmont Theile, the president, and Robert Miller, chairman of council, who had charge of proceedings. Two members of council were fathers of sons who faced appointment to the country. I had worked alongside Theile, the president, in a charitable organization and was on friendly terms with most of the other members of the council. In opening the debate of the proposed plan of allocation, the president advised the meeting that he and other members had met the director general who refused to alter the plan of appointments in any way and intended to hold the allocation meeting scheduled for the next morning. The representatives of the graduates had been kept up-to-date with plans by me, but they had failed to pass on the information to their fellows. There would be one compensation for Queenslanders going to the country hospitals. I had given my assurance that they would be transferred to the metropolitan hospitals for their second year if they so wished, thus placing them on an equal footing with their colleagues in the competition for posts in training of specialists. However, the president believed firmly that Queensland students were being discriminated against. This was the opinion of most present and finally the following resolutions were passed:

> 1. That the Director General be contacted tonight and told it is the opinion of Council that the proposed method of appointment of first year Resident Medical Officers to the Queensland Hospital Service is unacceptable to the profession. Council believes the meeting called for tomorrow morning should be deferred and that the southern graduates be included in the total pool with their results and that the posts should be awarded on merit. If any preference is to be shown it should be shown to the Queensland graduates.
> 2. That the Director General be informed that if he is unable to implement this request, he should be requested to defer any action on the appointments so that the Council may approach the Minister and the Premier, and also, if necessary, call a meeting of members employed in the Queensland Hospital Service to discuss what attitude they will adopt.

3. In the event of the Director General refusing to comply with either of these requests he be informed that Council intends to release its viewpoint to the press.

While the AMA council was meeting, I was dining with the Health minister at the Milano Restaurant. The minister had also invited Eric Saint, the dean of the faculty of Medicine, Douglas Gordon, professor of Social and Preventive Medicine, and Richard Strutton, the department's undersecretary, to discuss over dinner the establishment of community health centres in Queensland.

I returned home in convivial mood and retired for the night. In a few minutes the phone rang. The caller was Theile from the AMA wishing to read the resolutions the council had just passed. My mood changed as I listened. When the president had concluded, I reacted angrily. I said, "Monty, you and the AMA can jump in the lake," and replaced the receiver. A perplexed Theile returned to the meeting room and called aside the chairman, Robert Miller, and reported my reaction. The experienced Miller suggested that the council be told that the director general had not returned home from a meeting. This was done and the council began to discuss other business. Meanwhile I reflected on what I had said. I gradually realized I had erred. I decided to make amends by trying to contact Theile to discuss the subject more calmly. Fortunately the council meeting was still in progress when I rang. I suggested that I come to AMA House immediately to meet the council despite the late hour.

Around midnight at AMA House I explained the background to the decision, and my obligation to the country hospitals. I told them why the suggestion to consider the southern and the Queensland graduates as a group was impractible: there would be great difficulty comparing the results from several universities even if they were available. If such a suggestion were carried out I was still faced with the probability that southern graduates who might be allotted posts in the country would refuse to serve there. I confirmed my resolve to proceed with the allocation meeting on the Saturday morning, and left to allow the council to reconsider my comments. The minutes of the next discussion indicate a division of opinion among the councillors. Some were adamant that I had "sacrified principle for expediency" and wished the resolutions to stand. Others believed that the position would have to be accepted. Finally, the opinion of the latter group held sway and new resolutions were adopted. They read:

1. That in the light of discussion with the Director General implementation of Council's motions not be proceeded with.
2. That the Director General be written to in strong terms of protest at the method of selection where principles were sacrificed for expediency, and that he be requested to review the method to ensure that the same procedure was not employed next year.
3. That close contact be sought between the Director General, the students and the Australian Medical Association and the Association seek representation in future at the allotment of positions.
4. That the Director General be advised in writing of the previous motions of Council.

The council then instructed the president to give its views in a general way to the press. However, no statement from the president appeared in the weekend press.

On the Saturday morning the allocation meeting proceeded as scheduled. Two representatives of the Queensland graduates, Ian Gough and Robert Galley, accepted my invitation to be present and under my guidance they allocated one hundred Queenslanders to both city and country hospitals. After the meeting I made my way homeward believing I would have at least a temporary respite. It was not to be.

About 7 p.m., while taking coffee in my lounge the doorbell rang. The caller was John Ward, the president of the Princess Alexandra Hospital Resident Medical Association which had met that morning to discuss the subject. Ward handed me a copy of resolutions that had been passed at the meeting. They demanded that the director general rescind the allocations made that morning and that the Queenslanders all be posted to Brisbane hospitals. I invited Ward to discuss the resolutions over a cup of coffee during which I told him politely but firmly that I had no intention of acting in the way requested. However I agreed to meet the residents on Monday evening. At 5 p.m. on 30 November I faced approximately one hundred hostile residents and registrars in the Princess Alexandra Hospital lecture theatre. The doctors had come not only from that hospital but also from the other metropolitan hospitals, and Southport, Ipswich and Toowoomba. Once again I outlined the events leading up to the decision and invited the meeting to put forward any other practical way of obtaining new doctors for the country. The ensuing discussion produced no solution for finding country medical staff but many demands to allow all Queenslanders to work in Brisbane. After considerable time John Ward moved from the chair a vote of no confidence in the director general. He waited in vain for a colleague to second his motion. Eventually, Barbara Bain, a medical registrar at Princess Alexandra Hospital, addressed the meeting. She said she understood the director general's obligation to staff all hospitals but disagreed with his method of achieving it. However, as all discussion on the subject seemed to have been exhausted, she suggested the meeting terminate. With one or two exceptions, all present favoured the action suggested and the doctors dispersed. This was the last outward show of opposition.

The new doctors were expected to take up their appointments on 4 January 1971. Over the next few weeks, I made discreet enquiries regarding the intentions of Queenslanders posted to country hospitals. I learnt of no intended defections nor did I receive any notice from the southern graduates that they did not intend to come to Queensland. It was with some anxiety that I went to my office on 4 January to await reports from both the Brisbane and country superintendents, but with one or two exceptions all the graduates had commenced duty. The plan had succeeded in assuring staff numbers in all hospitals. In a few weeks I wrote to all the Queensland graduates asking if they wished to be considered for transfer to Brisbane if their former colleagues who failed the previous November examination were successful in the supplementary examinations. Only one application was received. The remainder had already realized the advantage of greater practical experience in the provincial hospitals. Some were already performing surgical operations under supervision that would be denied their Brisbane colleagues for many months. At the end of 1971, several of those who served in the country for the first year elected to stay there for another year despite assured posts in the metropolitan hospitals. Some of them continued with their training and later entered the ranks of specialists in various fields of medicine.

When Milan Brych Came to Queensland

To most Australians a Pacific island means a place to visit on vacation. In 1977, however, some began visiting one island for a far more serious purpose. They were seeking a cure for cancer at a clinic conducted by Milan Brych at Rarotonga, in the Cook Islands, about two thousand kilometres northeast of New Zealand. The patients included some for whom orthodox medicine could do no more. Urged on by relatives and friends to leave no stone unturned in a search for a miracle cure they were making the journey despite the consternation, perhaps the disapproval, of their previous medical attendants. Among the pilgrims were Queenslanders who had exhausted the facilities of the state's free hospital scheme to no avail. Accompanied by relatives, they were now spending up to $16,000 on fares, motel expenses and treatment at the island clinic. In many instances this money had been raised by public subscription. Only a small portion of these costs were recouped through medical benefits schemes. All who returned spoke highly of Brych, whose charm had instilled great confidence. Many claimed that the course of injections that he administered had produced marked improvement. The ability to walk had been restored in some who had been brought to the island on a stretcher.

The return of improved patients was followed by much publicity and roused great controversy. To many, the improvement in patients who had been given no hope of recovery by their regular doctors meant only one thing — Brych had a secret formula. Weight was given to this hypothesis by Brych himself in his continued refusal to reveal details of his treatment. The medical profession, particularly in the southern states of Australia, was sceptical. It was pointed out that remissions were not uncommon in the course of the disease no matter what treatment was given and that the improvements in Brych's patients were temporary only. Certain sections of the media openly supported the Cook Islands therapist, encouraging the idea that he had discovered a remedy unknown to the medical world. Nigel Gray, director of the Anti-Cancer Council of Victoria and Frank Quill, chief of staff on the *Melbourne Truth*, used the columns of the *Medical Journal of*

Australia to air opposing views. Gray claimed Brych was not medically qualified and that his theory was primitive nonsense. The Melbourne physician stated that of twenty-nine Victorian cases who had received much publicity in the press in previous months, fifteen had now died. In reply, Quill stated that senior journalists had found evidence to support Brych's claims of high survival rates after his treatment and regretted that Dr Gray made statements without first-hand knowledge of Brych's theory and competence.

The Queensland medical profession was publicly rather cautious in its approach to the controversy. Daniel Hart, president of the Queensland branch of the Australian Medical Association, said that Brych should be given a fair hearing on his treatment in Australia. While doctors were willing to discuss the subject in a general manner, there was less enthusiasm to appear on television programmes in which returned patients testified to the success of the Brych treatment. The medicos declined to tell a patient buoyed up by hope that such hope was false, that any improvement was temporary only, and that deterioration was inevitable.

During the controversy, Llew Edwards, a general practitioner and Queensland minister for Health (now Sir Llew), wrote twice to Brych asking him for details of his treatment and his results so that an evaluation of his method could be made in Queensland hospitals. As before, neither request was answered. Unlike members of the medical profession throughout the world who publish such matters for the benefit of others, Brych was silent. The minister had greater success when he approached the New Zealand medical authorities. From material forwarded by the Medical Council of New Zealand and Professor P.J. Scott of the Auckland School of Medicine an interesting story emerged.

Vlastimil (Milan) Brych was one of a number of Czechoslovakian refugees accepted by the New Zealand government in 1968. He claimed that he was a qualified medical practitioner but had not a single piece of evidence to support his claim. He was given a position in the pathology laboratory at the Auckland Hospital and spent much of his time polishing up on medical knowledge and writing up sections of textbooks. A thesis which he claimed had earned him a doctorate of philosophy in his native land was later found to be a series of paragraphs from these textbooks. In 1969, a sympathetic medical council granted him provisional registration as a medical practitioner and he was appointed a junior resident medical officer. Although Brych rarely wrote case notes on his patients and often displayed great ignorance, he was excused by reason of his background. His poor showing in the hospital wards did not prevent his full registration which was followed by an appointment in the Department of Radiotherapy where cancer patients were treated. Soon his name appeared often in the media and the public gained the impression that he was a brilliant scientist who had fled his country for political reasons. Although he was a full-time employee of the Auckland Hospital board he began treating patients privately and let it be known that he was conducting important research. It was discovered later that the only equipment that his research laboratory contained was a double bed. By 1972, Brych had appeared on a television programme claiming his outstanding success in the treatment of one type of cancer. His claims were based on the work at the radiotherapy centre where he was only a junior member of the staff. By this time he was attracting many private patients including many Australians. However, his behaviour and lack of knowledge, apparent to the Auckland specialists, brought an enquiry into Auckland cancer services. Professor Douglas Wright of Melbourne, who conducted the enquiry, said Brych was a "professional fibber" and Brych was held in contempt of the enquiry. These findings and further evidence from overseas resulted in Brych's deregistration by the medical council. He appealed and was reinstated pending the hearing. While Brych had offended the medical profession he still had many supporters among the lay public. A fund was opened to pay the legal expenses for his appeal. Erroneous claims were made that he had qualified in New Zealand and that he held specialist status. During this period he continued to treat private patients.

The medical council sent Professor Scott overseas to gather evidence to be presented when the appeal was heard. During visits to America, Italy and Czechoslovakia, Scott interviewed Brych's former wife, a previous neighbour, school teachers, scientists and university and medical staff at the institutions where he had claimed he had studied medicine and worked after graduating. Lists of graduates, scientific literature and court records were studied. When Scott returned to New Zealand the material collected revealed the following story.

Brych had a bright record at primary school but did not complete the necessary examination for entry to university. He served two prison terms for criminal offences. After the first imprisonment he was employed in a medical laboratory in an attempt at rehabilitation but was dismissed for faking results. No member of the medical school or institution knew him and scientists with whom he said that he had shared research facilities had never heard of him. One prison term covered the period in which he was supposed to have attended medical school. Shortly after this evidence was lodged with the New Zealand Supreme Court for the expected hearing, Brych withdrew his appeal and transferred his clinic to the Cook Islands.

Queensland's premier, Joh Bjelke-Petersen (now Sir Joh), firmly believed that the Cook Islands therapist had something to offer sufferers, and over several months endeavoured to have Brych visit the state. At last he was successful and a date was set for the visit. Brych was granted a permit to enter Australia by Malcolm McKellar, the commonwealth minister for Immigration, on the understanding that he did not treat patients nor practise medicine. However, McKellar had assured Brych that this restriction did not preclude him from having private discussions with members of the medical profession or from undertaking public engagements to expound his theories. The premier advised Llew Edwards, the minister for Health, that Brych would be willing to discuss his treatment with Brisbane specialists. At that time I was the director general of health and medical services in the state government. Two days prior to the date set down for Brych's arrival, Edwards and I met Warren Hastings, a general medical practitioner from Melbourne to whom the premier had referred some Queenslanders for subsequent treatment by the Czech. Hastings was one of the few practitioners who supported Brych and was making arrangements for the visit. He also assured us that we would be able to put questions to Brych. Accordingly on 31 March 1978 a number of Brisbane experts from related fields in cancer waited in the Executive Building, Brisbane, for the meeting. Of suave appearance and neatly attired in a trendy way, Brych entered the conference room with the premier accompanied by Warren Hastings and Ian Cleland, chairman of the Friends of Rarotonga Association. Prior to the meeting, the minister for Health had arranged that the approach would be to regard the visitor as having something to give the profession which it wished to evaluate. There would no reference to Bryce's personal history nor to any of the evidence collected by the New Zealand medical council.

In the opening stages of the two-hour discussion that followed, the premier said that Brych had just told him that a symposium should be arranged to which overseas visitors on cancer should be invited. However, the premier considered that a symposium was

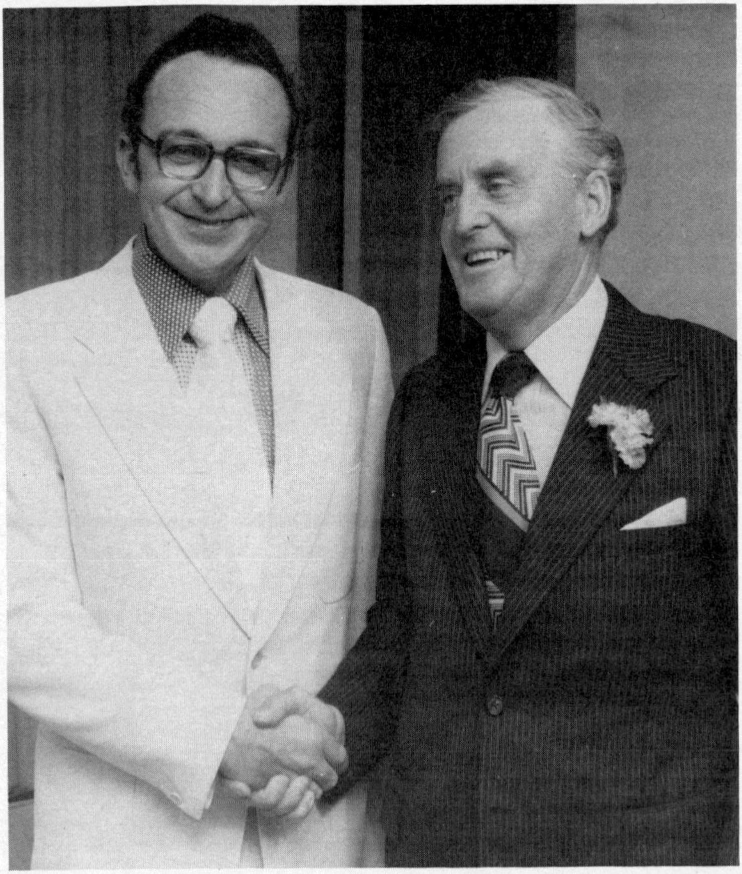

Cancer therapist Milan Brych was welcomed to Queensland by the premier, (now Sir) Joh Bjelke-Petersen in 1978. (Courtesy the *Courier-Mail*)

a matter for the future and he would like the meeting to proceed by the group asking questions; he hoped it would progress to the stage where agreement would be reached about starting a Brych clinic. The visitor was then invited to address the meeting but said that he preferred to be asked questions. Warren Hastings then asked Milan exactly what his treatment involved.

Speaking in fluent English with a very slight European accent, Brych used many medical terms and referred to several diagnostic and treatment procedures relating to cancer. However, he evaded any deep discussion on the subject and flatly refused to give any details of his treatment despite being pressed by several of those present. Ken Donald, the director of the Royal

Brisbane Hospital Department of Pathology, after unsuccessful attempts to induce the therapist to explain one particular process, claimed that the depth Brych reached, but beyond which he would not advance, could be attained by a high school student. Although the premier and Warren Hastings had given assurances that the Cook Islands therapist would answer questions, and Brych himself at the beginning of the meeting had invited questions, no definite reply emerged at any time. He claimed that the *Medical Journal of Australia* had published slanderous, lying statements about him and the present group was ridiculing him. He further alleged that attempts were being made to induce him to break the promise that he given the Immigration minister not to practise medicine while in Australia, despite the fact that he had been assured that such discussion was quite within the conditions under which he had been granted entry into the country. Towards the end of the meeting the premier stated that he was not going to accept the responsibility of letting something of this nature go when all that was being discussed was the question of Brych's doing in Queensland what he had been doing in New Zealand. This remark was followed by an interesting debate between the premier and Daniel Hart from the Australian Medical Association on the subject of divulging medical discoveries. The record of this reads as follows:

Dr Hart:	Mr Premier, it is quite obvious that you believe Dr Brych has something.
Premier:	I do believe that he gets some results on patients.
Dr Hart:	You do believe he has something?
Premier:	Yes.
Dr Hart:	Well, do you think he should tell us?
Premier:	Well cer. . . first of all, I have a few patents to my name.
Dr Hart:	Do you think he should tell us now tonight, sir? Do you think he should tell us what he has got?
Premier:	Here again, discussing it with Warren from time to time, over the last years Warren has said to me, it's not as simple as that.
Dr Hart:	Don't you think he should tell us what he has got, Mr Premier?
Premier:	Well, fair enough in some respects. Dr Hastings had said and Dr what's-his-name has said he is concerned with his patients and his documents and do this and that.
Dr Hart:	Don't you think he should tell us here and now, Sir?
Dr Edwards:	Mr Premier, I wonder if I could interrupt. I think we have had a fair go.

Premier: Just, just I would like to answer this one. I was just going to say I have had some patents patented and machines sold in earlier days, I have, first of all I spent years getting, building and building and developing this machine. I didn't go running around telling everybody exactly what I did. I know. . .

Dr Hart: Do you think he should keep a secret then, sir?

Premier: I believe that he has got every justification.

Dr Hart: In keeping it a secret?

Premier: No, to confirm exactly what he is doing it and improve on the methods and so on that he is doing. That he knows he, well I think he knows now, but until he has got, well his documentation ready: He has told me that by October Warren has told me that they should be ready.

Dr Hart: What about tonight? What about tonight?

Premier: Why should he tonight tell exactly what. . .

Dr Edwards: Mr Premier . . .

Dr Hart: Why shouldn't he?

Premier: Why should he?

Dr Edwards: Mr Premier, I wonder if I could interrupt.

Dr Hart: Yes.

Premier: Well why should he anyway?

Dr Hart: Because the whole. . . [inaudible].
Doctors in the world. . . [inaudible].

Premier: You wouldn't believe it anyway. You wouldn't believe it anyway.

Dr Edwards: I don't think that's going to get anywhere.

Premier: All we'll do. . . All we do. . . All I'll tell you I'm behind that man.

Over the next four days Brych's visit made headline news on the front pages of the press and featured largely on television programmes. Under headings on successive days in the *Courier-Mail* which read "JOH WANTS CANCER CLINIC HERE" and "BRYCH: I'LL OPEN BRISBANE CLINIC", the premier announced that Milan Brych might set up a clinic in Brisbane within two months and Brych stated emphatically that he would open such a clinic. The premier envisaged that the clinic would become the centre of world attention. Brych stated that the prior condition of his being registered by the Medical Board of Queensland was an absolute certainty. As events turned out no application for registration was made but had it been placed before the board, it would certainly have been rejected. To obtain such recognition it would have been necessary for Brych to produce evidence that he held a degree in medicine equal to that awarded in Queensland and pass a further examination conducted in Australia. Although he had referred to his Czechoslovakian and New Zealand degrees, evidence from the New Zealand medical council revealed that he held neither and the specialists who attended the Executive Building meeting were adamant that he did not possess sufficient knowledge to pass the required examination. During a television interview the therapist gave yet another reason for his refusal to discuss his treatment. He stated that by asking simple questions he discovered that members of the panel of doctors he had met did not possess even the very, very basic terminological knowledge to discuss the subject.

Press reports indicated that Dr Llew Edwards did not share the premier's enthusiasm for the Cook Islands therapist. He was expected to report to cabinet that Brych had nothing to offer and the media predicted a headlong clash between the premier and his minister for Health. Reports of the cabinet meeting suggested that the premier was out on a limb over his personal support for the visiting therapist. When Dr Edwards indicated that he intended to make a statement in parliament he was encouraged by all the other ministers except the premier, who insisted that it be written into the minutes that Dr Edwards should do so as Health minister and not as government policy. When parliament assembled the next day, the political overtones associated with the expected statement drew a packed gallery where there was standing room only. The minister told a hushed parliament that he was not convinced that Brych should be encouraged to establish a clinic in Queensland. As he made this remark, the premier sat in the ministerial front bench shaking his head. Edwards claimed that Brych had little or no medical knowledge, and that he "appeared totally incapable of discussing technically or scientifically even the simplest of medical and laboratory techniques". The statement was accompanied by the tabling of documents that included reports from the Medical Council of New Zealand, a transcript of a recording of the meeting with Brych at the Executive Building and other relevant material.

A *Courier-Mail* editorial had this to say:

HEALTH MINISTER ON MR BRYCH

> It is time, now, to take the Brych affair out of politics and put it back where it belongs, in the tribunals of medicine.
>
> Yesterday the State Health Minister (Dr Edwards), in conflict with the Premier, made clear where the Health Department stands on Milan Brych, Cook Islands cancer therapist. Dr Edwards told Parlia-

ment that Mr Brych's main asset was a near-hypnotic charm, but that he had "nothing new to offer Queenslanders in cancer therapy".

Dr Edwards' much-heralded statement gave the considerable number of people who have become "Brych-watchers" little new information, but probably confirmed many judgements.

In a general condemnation he said that Mr Brych administered drugs in "an unscientific and often fatal combination." The Premier was unimpressed and unrepentant. It seems he genuinely cannot conceive despite the mass of material tabled by Dr Edwards, why there should be suspicions about Mr Brych.

Mr Bjelke-Petersen still wants Mr Brych to set up a cancer clinic in Brisbane. If he is qualified, he should be free to do so. But is Mr Brych qualified?

This is not a matter for politicians to decide, least of all the Premier. If Mr Brych wants to practise in Queensland he must ask the Medical Board of Queensland for registration as a medical practitioner.

That is the body to which the law of Queensland has given the responsibility of protecting Queenslanders from quackery. It consists of some of the State's eminent medical men and is above political patronage.

If what Dr Edwards revealed yesterday is correct, obviously Mr Brych has no chance of gaining registration. It is unlikely he will even try, despite the Premier's confidence.

JOH'S ATTITUDE

Mr Bjelke-Petersen's attitude to Mr Brych has been that of Medici patron with a new artist.

He seems to believe that he is presenting a genius who has discovered secrets which all the cancer programmes of the world, helped by great minds and funded by thousands of millions of dollars have failed to do.

The Premier's Brych crusade has made him look foolish. If Mr Bjelke-Petersen is capable of making such irrational and interfering decisions in the Brych affair, Government members must wonder about his decisions on other matters.

Not long after his visit to Queensland, Brych left the Cook Islands for America where he commenced new operations. A press report of 1 October 1982 said that he faced eighteen charges in California including criminal conspiracy, grand theft by false pretences, feloniously practising medicine without a licence and various violations of the cancer control statues. On 28 July 1983 the Los Angeles Superior Court sentenced him to six years' jail. Llew Edwards's stand was vindicated.

References

Abbreviations

ADB	*Australian Dictionary of Biography*. Melbourne: Melbourne University Press.
AMA	Australian Medical Association.
AMG	*Australasian Medical Gazette.*
AMJ	*Australian Medical Journal.*
AONSW	Archives Office of New South Wales.
BC	*Brisbane Courier.*
CM	*Courier-Mail*, Brisbane.
MBC	*Moreton Bay Courier.*
MJA	*Medical Journal of Australia.*
ML	Mitchell Library, Sydney.
NSWGG	*New South Wales Government Gazette.*
OML	Oxley Memorial Library, Brisbane.
QGG	*Queensland Government Gazette.*
QPD	*Queensland Parliamentary Debates.*
QPP	*Queensland Parliamentary Papers.*
QSA	Queensland State Archives.
V&P	*Queensland Legislative Assembly Votes and Proceedings.*
SAPP	*South Australia Parliamentary Papers.*
TEL	*Telegraph*, Brisbane.

1. Surgeon Sacked in Sex Scandal

Bigge, J.T. Report into the colony of New South Wales. And Appendix. 1822, ML.

Court of enquiry, Brisbane Town, 21 November 1832. 4/2204.1, AONSW.

HM General Hospital, Moreton Bay. Records. HOS 1/6, 1/10, 1/11, QSA.

Letter from Bowman to McLeay, 15 December 1832. 4/2204.1, AONSW.

______. J.F. Murray to Anna Bunn, 10 May 1830. AM, 63/7, ML.

Russell, H.S. *Genesis of Queensland*. Appendix E. Sydney: Turner and Henderson, 1888.

Spicer, P. Spicer's Diary, OML.

2. Death's *Emigrant*

Correspondence between Captain Wickham and colonial secretary's department. Microfilm A/2.21, frames 663-784, OML.
HM General Hospital, Moreton Bay (Brisbane Hospital). Records. HOS 1/4, 1/7, 1/12, 1/13, 1/15, 1/G1, 1/G2, 1/G3, 1/D2, QSA.
Lang, J.D. *Cooksland in North Eastern Australia.* London: Longmans, 1847.
MBC. 1847–50, especially August–October 1850.

3. Moreton Bay's First Anaesthetist

Belisario, John C. "Belisario, John". In *ADB* 3, 1851–90, p. 132.
Brisbane Hospital. Records. HOS 1/7, f. 252. HOS 1/25, f. 164, QSA.
Craig, C. "Pugh, William Russ". In *ADB* 2, 1788–1850, p. 355.
MBC. 20 January, 16 May, 10 November 1849; 14 June 1851; 26 August 1854.
MJA. 1 (1923): 381.
Robinson, Victor. *The Story of Medicine*. New York: New Home Library, 1943.

4. Love and Blindness

Executive Council. Minutes, vol. 4, 1862. EXE/D28, QSA.
Judge Lutwyche. Colonial secretary in-letters. 61/2754, QSA.
MBC. 12 May 1860; 2 April 1861.
Petitions from Maryborough and Wide Bay, and Musket Flat to the governor. Colonial secretary in-letters. 61/2863, QSA.

5. The Unusual Dr Jonathan Labatt

BC. 10 January 1866.
Correspondence on Labatt's release. Colonial secretary in-letters. 62/1643, QSA.
Glennie, B. Australian Diary of Reverend Benjamin Glennie, 16 January 1848 to 30 September 1860. Typescript 5 November 1854, OML.
Letters from Labatt to Bowen, 5 July 1862. Colonial secretary in-letters. 62/1711, QSA.
______. Labatt to colonial secretary, 7 March 1866. Colonial secretary in-letters. 66/1519, QSA.
______. Labatt to Herbert; 8 March 1862. Colonial secretary in-letters. 62/756, QSA.
______. Labatt to Manning, 26 February 1862. Colonial secretary in-letters. 62/675, QSA.

______. McDonald to colonial secretary, 21 February 1866. Colonial secretary in-letters. 66/1519, QSA.
MBC. 7 April, 11 August 1855; 6 June 1857.
NSWGG 31 (18 May 1852): 829.
______. 35 (24 June 1854): 184.
QGG 6 (26 August 1865): 735.
Report of the select committee on Dr Labatt. *V&P* (1864): 1283.

6. Birth of a Hospital

Brisbane Hospital. Letters from committee secretary. HOS 1/G1, QSA.
______. Minutes of committee meetings. Series HOS 1/D2-HOS 1/D8, QSA.
______. Registers of cases and treatment. HOS 1/7, 1/25, QSA.
Executive Council. Minute, 31 December 1863. EXE/E8, QSA.
Letter from Colonial Secretary R.G.W. Herbert to Brisbane Hospital committee, 15 April 1864. 64/324, COL/R4, QSA.
______. 2 April 1864. 64/265, COL/R4, QSA.
Letter from Manning, principal undersecretary, colonial secretary's department, to Brisbane Hospital committee, 2 September 1862. 62/530, COL/R3, QSA.
______. 4 May 1865. 65/300, COL/R4, QSA.
______. 3 June 1865. 65/393, COL/R4, QSA.
MBC. 1847–67.
Moreton Bay Benevolent Society. Minutes. 1/D1, QSA.

7. Gulf Fever

Elkington, J.S.C. "Quarantine in Queensland". *AMG* 31 (1912): 433.
"Historical and Geographical Survey of Part of North Australia". CSIRO Divisional Report 59/2.
James, P. "Remarks on the Fevers and Diseases of Northern Queensland". *AMG* 10 (1891): 300.
Landsborough, W. Journal of Expedition from Carpentaria in Search of *Burke and Wills*. Melbourne: Watson and MacKinnon, 1862.
Letters from A.C. Gregory. *SAPP* 3, No. 170 of 1861.
Palmer, E. *Early Days in North Queensland*. Sydney: Angus and Robertson, 1903.
Stokes, J.L. *Discoveries in Australia*. Reprinted by Libraries Board of South Australia, 1969.
Sutherland, G. *Pioneering Days — Thrilling Incidents*. Brisbane: W.H. Wendt and Co., 1913.
Weekly-Herald. 7 July, 4 August 1866.
White, J.A. "The Fevers of the Gulf of Carpentaria". *AMJ* 12 (1867): 361.

8. The Case of the Missing Head

Australasian. 3 June 1922.

BC. 11, 12, 15, 16, 28 November 1867; 17, 26, 31 March, 16 May, 8, 20 June 1868.

Bird, J.T.S. *The Early History of Rockhampton*. Rockhampton: Morning Bulletin, 1904.

McDonald, Lorna. *Rockhampton — A History of the City and Districts*. Brisbane: University of Queensland Press, 1981.

Morrison, A.A. "Griffin, Thomas John Augustus". In *ADB* 4, 1851–90, p. 300.

QGG 9 (12 June 1868): 581.

Rockhampton Bulletin and Central Queensland Advertiser. 9 Novermber 1867; 19, 21 March, 2, 4, 6, 9, 11, 13 June 1868.

Salter, Elizabeth. *Daisy Bates*. New York: Coward, McCann and Geoghegan, 1972.

9. Snakes in the Asylum

BC. 17 May 1869.

Darvall evidence. Report of select committee on Dr Labatt. *V&P* (1864): 1287.

Knight, J.J. *In the Early Days*. Brisbane: Sapsford and Co., 1895.

Letter from Challinor to colonial secretary, 30 March 1870. COL A139, 70/962, QSA.

______. J. Meade Swift to colonial secretary, 30 May 1863. COL A40, 63/1169, QSA.

______. Labatt to colonial secretary, 5 July 1862. COL A40, 62/1711, QSA.

______. W.A. Brown to colonial secretary, 17 July 1863. COL A42, 63/1591, QSA.

______. William Ewington to Governor Bowen, 7 September 1863. COL A44, 63/2050, QSA.

QPD 9 (1869): 155.

Queensland Times. 1, 3 December 1868; 5 January 1869.

Report of the select committee on the hospitals of the colony. *V&P* (1866): 1605.

V&P (1866): 673.

______. 2 (1867): 1063.

______. (1868–69): 687.

______. 1 (1869): 905.

10. Brisbane Brothels

BC. 26 JUly 1881; 22, 23 October 1867; 13, 14 January 1868.

Hobbs, W. "Report of the working of The Act for the Prevention of Contagious Disease". *V&P* 2 (1879): 1273.
Home secretary's correspondence. HOM/J80, 1911/7759; HOM/J80, 1907/10380, QSA.
Petition on "The Act for the Prevention of Contagious Diseases". *V&P* 3 (1884): 1167.
QGG 47 (24 August 1911): 591.
QPD 44 (1884): 523.
______. 50 (1886): 1045.
Queensland Figaro. 17 October 1885, p. 614.

11. From Convict to Doctor

Brisbane Age. 2 July 1905.
Cullen, J.H. *Young Ireland in Exile*. Dublin: Talbot Press, 1928.
Hodges, J.G. *Report of the Proceedings under the Treason Felony Act, Commission Court, Dublin, August and October 1848*. Dublin: Alex Thom, 1848.
Irish Tribune. 1848.
Kiernan, T.J. *The Irish Exiles in Australia*. Dublin: Clonmire and Reynolds, 1954.
McLay, Y.M. *James Quinn, First Catholic Bishop of Brisbane*. Armadale, Victoria: Graphic Books, 1979.
Melbourne Argus. 24 July 1854.
Mitchel, John. *Jail Journal*. Dublin: M.H. Gill and Son, n.d.
Nesbitt, Caroline. Great-great-granddaughter of O'Doherty. Interview with author. North Sandwich, New Hampshire, USA, April 1982.
O'Doherty Papers. National Library of Ireland, Dublin.
O'Doherty speeches in Queensland parliament. *QPD* 1867–73 and 1877–85.
Poems by Eva of the Nation. Dublin: M.H. Gill and Son, 1909.
Queensland Times. 7 March, 12 August 1862; 24 July 1863.
Records of Irish state prisoners. Convict papers, 1849. Tasmanian Archives.

12. Tinkering in the Bush

BC. "The Murder of Simon Ziemon". 18 December 1871; 14 May 1872.
QPD 12 (1871–72).

13. Governor in Waiting

Boyce, Peter. "Kennedy, Sir Arthur Edward". In *ADB* 5, 1851–90, p. 15.
BC. 27 March, 2, 11, 19 April 1877.

14. Typhoid at Toowoomba

Report of the board appointed to investigate the cause of the prevalence of typhoid fever at Toowoomba. *V&P* 2 (1878): 767.

Telegram from W.H. Groom to colonial secretary, 24 April 1884. COL/A388, 1884/3112, QSA.

15. Too Drunk To Operate

BC. 30 May, 3, 4, 6, 11, 14 June 1878.

Brisbane Hospital committee meeting. Minutes, 29 May 1878. HOS 1/D10, QSA.

16. "Horsewhip the Doctor"

CM. 30 December 1947.

Dods, Lorimer. "Early Pediatrics in the Antipodes". *MJA* 1 (1961): 841.

Hall, Peter. *A Century of Care*. Brisbane: Royal Children's Hospital (1878–1978).

Hospital for Sick Children. Annual report of 1890. Royal Brisbane Hospital Archives.

Mackerras, I.M. "Alfred Jefferis Turner and Amateur Entomology in Australia". Proceedings of the Royal Society of Queensland No. 7, vol. 60 (1948): 69. Contains an extensive bibliography of Turner's papers.

North Queensland Register. 18, 25 June 1900.

Obituary. *MJA* 1 (1948): 417.

Queensland Health department infant welfare division. Annual reports. *QPP* 1926–37.

Townsville Bulletin. 13 June 1900.

Turner, A. Jefferis. "Experiences in Preventive Medicine". *MJA* 2 (1938): 805.

______. "Infantile Mortality". *AMG* 29 (1910): 277.

______. "The Medical Ideal". *AMG* 26 (1907): 1.

______. "Report of Proceedings of International Congress on Tuberculosis, London, 1901". *QPP* 1 (1902): 905.

17. Leper Islands of Moreton Bay

Bancroft, J. "Leprosy in Queensland". *AMG* 11 (1892): 427.

BC. 12, 13 April 1892.

Brisbane Hospital. Register of cases and treatment. HOS 1/25, p. 258, QSA.

Cook, C. "The Epidemiology of Leprosy in Australia". Commonwealth Health department Service Publication No. 38.
QPD 67 (1892): 230.
QPP 2 (1908): 859.
_____. (1940): 1056.
_____. 2 (1960–61): 844.
_____ (1973–74): 1919.
Worker. 14 December 1895.

18. The First Woman

BC. 29 May, 24 December 1891; 29 May 1923.
Hospital for Sick Children. Annual reports 1896–1917. OML.
Lancet. 6 July 1861; 7 October 1865.
Leggett, C.A.C. "Cooper, Lilian Violet". In *ADB* 8, 1891–1939, p. 105.
Queenslander. 23 May 1891.
Queensland Medical Society. Minutes of meeting, 13 June 1893. AMA House, Brisbane.
Skewes, Edna M. *Life Comes to Newness*. Brisbane: Boolarong Press, 1982.
Summers, Harry. *They Crossed the River*. Brisbane: University of Queensland Press, 1979.

19. Black Death

BC. 19 January, 7 March, 29, 30 April, 1, 12, 16, 23 May 1900.
Cumpston, J.H.L. and F. McCallum. "The History of Plague in Australia". Commonwealth Health department Service Publication No. 32.
Halford, A.C.F. Report of plague in Brisbane, 1901–02. State Health Library.
Ham, B. Burnett. "Report of Plague in Queensland, 1900–07". *QPP* 2 (1907): 59.

20. War Hysteria

BC. 6, 7 August 1914; 31 October 1919; 24, 26 August 1926.
British Medical Association (Queensland Branch). Minutes of meetings, 14 April (special), 23 April, 21 May 1915; 7 November 1919.
Daily Mail. 19 June 1920.
Daily Standard. 2 July 1914.
Hirschfeld, E. "Prevention of Infectious Diseases". Presented 13 August 1892. Proceedings of the Royal Society of Queensland vol. 9 (1892–93).

Interpreter's report on consular files; report on conspiracy against Mrs Hirschfeld; opinion of Chambers and McNab. Correspondence files – Dr E. Hirschfeld. B.P.4/1, item 66/4/891, Australian Archives, Brisbane.

Legett, C.A.C. "Hirschfeld, Eugen". In *ADB* 9, 1891–1939, p. 309.

Letter from Hirschfeld to general consul, Sydney, 27 July 1908; letter from Monash to Garran; report of aliens board; Garran's interrogation of Hirschfeld and the deportation recommendation. Attorney general's department, Dr Hirschfeld. A456, W8/4/129, Australian Archives, Canberra.

MJA 15, 22 November 1919; 7, 14 February, 24 April 1920.

QPD 118 (1914): 1404, 1443, 1656.

TEL. 28 January 1907; 6 May 1912.

21. The Bundaberg Tragedy

BC. 31 January, 1, 2, 3 February 1928.

"Report of Royal Commission of Inquiry into Fatalities at Bundaberg". Commonwealth Parliamentary Papers (1926–28): 1085.

22. Fraud or Medical Genius

Cilento, R.W. "Report of the Muscle Re-Education Clinic, Townsville (Sister Kenny)". PRE/A1101, 4708/34, QSA.

CM. 1 April 1935; 6 January 1938; 18 November 1947.

Cohn, Victor. *Sister Kenny.* Minneapolis: University of Minnesota Press, 1975.

Fryberg, Sir Abraham, former superintendent Kenny Clinic. Interview with author. Brisbane 1982.

Kenny, Elizabeth. (In collaboration with Martha Ostenso.) *And They Shall Walk.* New York: Dodd, Mead and Co., 1943.

McCracken, Mary, (nee Stewart-Kenny). Interview with author. Caloundra, Queensland, 1982.

Obituary. *British Medical Journal* (6 December 1952): 1262.

Pye, Aubrey. Interview with author. Brisbane, 1982.

QPP 2 (1947–48): 1021.

Queenslander. 3 April 1930.

"Report of the Royal Commission to Enquire into the Treatment of Infantile Paralysis". *MJA* 1 (29 January 1938): 187.

Summary of facts leading to the establishment of Sister Kenny Clinic. Queensland Health department records.

Toowoomba Chronicle. 1 December 1952.

Townsville Daily Bulletin. 6 October 1936.

23. A Short Funeral

Lack, Clem. *Three Decades of Queensland Political History, 1929–1960*. Brisbane: Government Printer, n.d.
QPD 251 (1969–70): 458.

24. The Country Needs You

AMA council meeting. Minutes, 27 November 1970. AMA House.
CM. 27 November 1970.
QPD 252 (1970): 2322, 2474.

25. When Milan Brych Came to Queensland

CM. 1, 3, 4, 5 April 1978; 29 July 1983. Documents tabled by Dr L.R. Edwards (later Sir Llewellyn) in Queensland parliament, 4 April 1978. No. 150 (a-k).
Gray, Nigel. "Milan Brych and the Medical Profession". *MJA* 2 (1978): 195.
QPD 274 (1978): 54.
Sunday Mail, Brisbane. 2 April 1978.
TEL. 31 March, 1, 3, 4 April 1978; 1 October 1982; 28 July 1983.